Powering health

A complete guide to nutrition and supplement

Dr. Lily O. Walker

© [Dr. Lily O. Walker] [2024]

Table of Contents

Introduction

In a time when pursuing a holistic approach to health has become critical, "Powering Health: A Comprehensive Guide to Nutrition and Supplements" is an invaluable resource for achieving peak vitality. Readers are welcomed on a trip that goes beyond traditional health guidelines in this revolutionary examination of the complex link between nutrition and supplements, which offers a deep knowledge of how our dietary and supplement choices may have a tremendous influence on our general well-being. The need to maintain a nutritious and well-balanced diet becomes more and more evident as we manage the difficulties of contemporary living. "Powering Health" aims to provide readers with information that goes beyond fads and trends by demystifying the world of nutrition and supplements. This book is intended to be your reliable companion whether you are a seasoned health enthusiast or someone starting a fresh wellness journey. It offers a road map for navigating the confusing array of dietary options and supplements that are now on the market. This book explores the science behind nutrition and supplements, dispelling the myths around them, rather than just providing a list of dietary dos and don'ts. "Powering Health" gives readers the knowledge and skills to make choices that are specific to their requirements, preferences, and health objectives. It is supported by the most recent research and professional perspectives.

The book's comprehensive approach recognizes that diet may have a significant influence on mental health in addition to physical health. A careful combination of case studies, practical guidance, and doable tasks leads readers toward the goal of obtaining a state of balanced health that includes mental and physical well-being. "Powering Health" is more than simply a manual; it's a travel companion that offers the wisdom and motivation required to make long-lasting and significant adjustments. Turn the pages to uncover the transformational potential for a healthier, more vibrant, and empowered life that is contained within your daily supplement regimen and food choices.

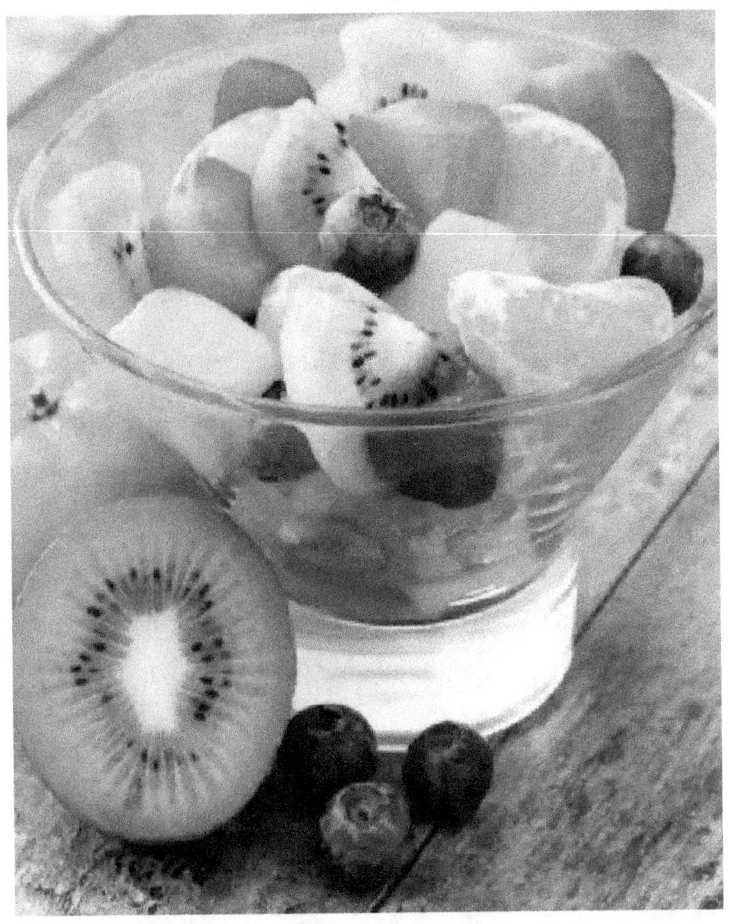

Chapter 1: Comprehending Nutrition

The foundation of a healthy and happy existence is proper nutrition. It is essential for sustaining general health, fostering development, and averting several illnesses. Comprehending the basic concepts of nutrition entails knowing how our bodies use the foods that we eat. This thorough book tries to clarify the significance of nutrition, the essential elements that our bodies need, and the process of making wise decisions for a healthy, well-balanced diet.

1. The Foundations of Diet: The process by which our bodies get and use the materials required for development, upkeep, and energy is known as nutrition. Micronutrients and macronutrients are two of the fundamental elements of nutrition.

- Macronutrients:- Carbohydrates: Found in grains, fruits, and vegetables, they are the main source of energy.

- Proteins: Found in meat, dairy, and plant-based foods, proteins are necessary for tissue development and repair.

- Fats: Found in oils, nuts, and seeds; essential for storing energy and absorbing fat-soluble vitamins.

- Micronutrients:- Vitamins: Essential for many body processes, including metabolism and immunological support.

- Minerals: Vital for neuron function, bone health, and fluid balance.

2. The Value of a Well-Balanced Diet: The body gets the proper amount of nutrients from a balanced diet to perform at its best.

This entails combining a range of meals from many dietary categories, such as whole grains, fruits, vegetables, lean meats, and healthy fats. Maintaining excellent health requires limiting one's intake of processed foods, sweets, and saturated fats.

3. Energy Balance and Caloric Intake: Comprehending the equilibrium between energy expenditure and intake is essential for managing body weight. A calorie shortfall causes weight reduction, but consuming more calories than the body requires causes weight gain. Two essential elements of controlling calorie intake are portion management and macronutrient balance.

4. **Nutritional Guidelines:** Dietary guidelines, which propose food kinds and quantities to enhance health and avoid chronic illnesses, are available in many nations. These recommendations often stress how crucial it is to:

- Consuming a range of foods high in nutrients. Reducing the use of salt, added sugars, and saturated fats. Drinking water is your main hydration source.

5. **Diet and Particular Medical Conditions:** There may be circumstances and life stages that call for certain dietary concerns. For instance, specific diet programs may be required for athletes, chronic sickness patients, and expectant mothers. Personalized advice may be obtained by speaking with licensed dietitians or other medical specialists.

6. The Significance of Hydration: One of the main components of nutrition is getting enough water. Digestion, nutrition absorption, temperature control, and general cellular function all depend on water. It is advised to drink the right quantity of water each day, depending on one's requirements and degree of activity.

Knowing nutrition is about giving your body the proper mix of nutrients to support optimum health, not only about counting calories. One may start on the path to a better and more satisfying life by making educated food choices, eating a balanced diet, and being aware of their unique nutritional requirements. Always keep in mind that education, awareness, and a dedication to lifetime well-being are the keys to healthy eating.

1.1. Nutrition Fundamentals

"Unlocking Vitality: The Basics of Nutrition Unveiled," a fascinating investigation into the realm of nutrition, is your key to comprehending how the food you consume changes your well-being. Set off on a transforming path to radiant health and unlimited vitality. Prepare to learn the nutrition secrets that will enable you to make wise decisions for a healthy, happy life.

1. Taking Care of Your Body: The Fundamentals of Nutrition

Explore the basic ideas that are the basis of a healthy way of living. Discover how every mouthful adds to the health symphony within your body, from vital minerals to the importance of a balanced diet.

2. The Potency of Foods High in Nutrients
Discover the amazing variety of foods that are high in nutrients. Discover the rainbow of options that may improve your health and energy, from colorful fruits and vegetables to nutrient-dense grains and lean meats.

3. Harmony of Macronutrients: A Balancing Act
Learn about the intricate relationships between the three macronutrients—fats, proteins, and carbohydrates—and how each one affects your body's ability to produce

energy, support muscle function, and maintain overall energy levels.

4. Optimal Wellness: Micronutrients Beyond the Plate

Learn about the hidden heroes of nutrition: minerals and vitamins. Discover their vital functions in strengthening your bones and enhancing your immune system. Discover how to include nutrients into every food for a nutrient-rich lifestyle.

5. Elevate Your Hydration: The Energy Fountain

Satisfy your need for energy as you investigate the rejuvenating influence of water. Discover the benefits of being hydrated—a seemingly simple yet significant action that may promote digestion, maintain proper water balance, and improve cognitive performance.

6. Making Wise Decisions: The Practice of Mindful Eating

Learn how to limit portion sizes, analyze urges, and appreciate each mouthful as you become an expert in mindful eating. Transform each meal into a fulfilling experience that goes beyond simple nourishment to improve your relationship with food.

The Basics of Nutrition Unveiled" is your ticket to a robust, resilient, and energetic existence. Equipped with an understanding of the fundamentals of nutrition, you may design a way of living that not only satisfies your physical needs but also increases your energy level. Accept the road to a bright and happy life as you unleash vitality via the transformational power of diet. Begin your journey right now!

1.2 Macronutrients: Fats, Proteins, and Carbohydrates

Macronutrients are the main players in the complex dance of nutrition; they control the flow and ebb of energy in our bodies. The book "Fuel for Life: Unveiling the Power of Macronutrients" offers an insider's perspective on the vital functions of fats, proteins, and carbohydrates—the trinity of nutrients that keeps us going throughout the day. Let's explore the intriguing realm of macronutrients and learn how their interplay produces a symphony of life.

1. The Body's Preferred Fuel: Carbohydrates

Frequently referred to as the body's preferred energy source, carbohydrates power our everyday activities. Examine the two primary varieties—simple and complex—and learn how they affect blood sugar levels, offering either long-lasting endurance or short bursts of energy. Learn the truth about carbohydrates and bust any misconceptions that could have made your connection with this important macronutrient more difficult.

2. Proteins: The Components That Make Up Life

Enter the world of proteins, the creators of cellular repair and structure. Find more about the many functions they perform, including promoting immune system support and muscle development and repair. Learn about the benefits of consuming a range of protein sources and the beauty of both full and incomplete proteins.

3. Fats: More Than Just a Taste

Misunderstood, fat is a complex macronutrient that is essential for many body processes. Learn about the differences between saturated and unsaturated fats and their effects on hormone synthesis, cognitive function, and general energy storage. Discover the benefits of combining omega-3 and omega-6 fatty acids and discover how to get the right balance for your health.

4.   Identifying the Balance of Macronutrients

Set out on a quest to discover the precise ratio of fats, proteins, and carbs that suit your requirements and objectives. Find out how changing your intake of macronutrients may significantly impact your goals, whether you're an athlete looking to reach peak performance, a person trying to lose weight, or someone just trying to feel better overall.

5. Myth-busting and Useful Advice

Learn to avoid frequent misunderstandings about macronutrients and get useful advice on how to include a healthy mix in your regular meals. Gain the ability to choose foods, portion sizes, and meal scheduling wisely so that you can provide your body with the best possible nourishment.

1.3 Minerals and Vitamins as Micronutrients

Micronutrients are the exquisite conductors weaving the complex web of nourishment into our bodies' symphony of wellness. The book "Essential Elegance: Micronutrients Unveiled" is an invitation for you to take a voyage through the fascinating world of vitamins and minerals, the hidden heroes with significant impact on human health. Come explore the intricate dance of these micronutrients with us and learn about their vital roles in achieving optimum health.

1. The Magnificence of Vitamins: Keepers of Life

Vitamins are the little powerhouses that are necessary for so many different biological processes. Discover the many vitamin families, from the immune-stimulating Vitamin C to the bone-strengthening Vitamin D. Learn how to get these essential nutrients from a vibrant variety of fruits, vegetables, and other healthy foods. Discover the delicate balance necessary for maximum health.

2. The Enchantment of Minerals: Foundational Elements of Hardiness

The unsung heroes of strength, minerals are essential for nerve function, fluid balance regulation, and structural integrity. Explore the universe of minerals, including magnesium, calcium, iron, zinc, and zinc, and learn about their significant effects on enzymatic processes and bone health. Learn about the art of mineral synergy and how certain elements complement one another to promote general health.

3.   Dissecting Inadequacies and Achievements

Examine the effects of micronutrient imbalances by delving into the domains of excesses and deficiencies. Learn how an excess or deficiency of vitamins and minerals may cause a variety of health problems and how balance is necessary for long-term health.

4. Handling the Micronutrient Labyrinth

Set off on a journey of mindful eating and learn how to include a variety of nutrient-dense, high-quality meals into your regular diet. Learn useful advice for making sure you consume enough whole foods or, if needed, properly selected supplements to satisfy your daily requirements for micronutrients.

5. Micronutrients and Well-Being: An All-encompassing Perspective

Recognize how important vitamins and minerals are to general health. Examine the roles that these micronutrients play in mood management, cognitive function, and the body's defensive systems. Acknowledge a comprehensive perspective on nutrition that considers the complex dance of micronutrients as an essential component of the path to well-being.

Chapter 2: Constructing a Harmonious Plate

A balanced and healthful diet is something that often gets neglected in the rush of everyday life. But putting together a balanced meal is necessary for general health and energy. The body gets the vitamins, minerals, and nutrients it needs from a balanced plate to perform at its best. This article will examine the essential elements of a well-balanced plate and provide helpful advice for preparing a healthy and filling dinner.

The Basis of an Equilibrated Dish:

1. Serum: Protein is essential for immune system support, tissue growth and repair, and muscle mass maintenance. Add sources of lean protein such as fish, poultry, tofu, beans, and lentils. Try to eat no more than 25% of your plate or a quantity that suits your requirements.

2. Vegetables: Vegetables that are rich in color and nutrients should make up half of your dish. These provide vital minerals, vitamins, fiber, and antioxidants. To guarantee a wide spectrum of nutrients, include a variety of veggies, such as bell peppers, broccoli, carrots, and leafy greens.

3. Complete Grains: The high fiber content of whole grains facilitates better digestion and blood sugar regulation. Aim to fill around 25% of your plate with whole grains such as quinoa, brown rice, whole wheat, or oats. These grains add to a sensation of fullness and provide prolonged energy.

4. Healthy Fats: Add sources of good fats to your diet to help absorb fat-soluble vitamins and boost brain function. Include items in moderation such as avocados, almonds, seeds, and olive oil. Due to the high-calorie content of fats, watch how much you eat.

5. Dairy and Dairy Substitutes: Dairy products and their fortified counterparts are great providers of protein, calcium, and vitamin D. For general well-being and bone health, include a dish of plant-based alternatives, yogurt, or milk.

Help for Assembling a Well-Balanced Plate:

1. Control Point: Take note of serving sizes to prevent overindulging. Reduce the size of your dishes, bowls, and utensils to aid with portion management. Take note of your body's signals of hunger and fullness.

2. Diversity Is Essential: For a wide spectrum of nutrients, try to eat a variety of meals. To make your meals interesting and fulfilling, try various grains, veggies, proteins, and fats.

3. Conscientious Consumption: Chew gently, enjoying every taste. During meals, pay attention to your body's signals of hunger and fullness and stay away from distractions like television and cell phones.

This promotes conscious eating and aids in limiting intake.

4. Remain Hydrated: Water is necessary for good health in general. Stay hydrated by sipping water throughout the day. Hunger pangs may sometimes be indicators of dehydration.

5. Make a Plan: To make sure you have a range of nutrient-dense foods accessible, plan your meals. This might assist you in choosing better selections instead of grabbing for quick, less nourishing ones. Maintaining excellent health and well-being starts with building a balanced plate. You can support your body's demands and foster long-term health by consuming a range of nutrient-rich meals in sensible quantities. Recall that maintaining a balanced diet is about making educated decisions that fit your interests and way of life rather than following rigid guidelines. Begin modestly, adjust gradually, and enjoy the trip toward a more nutritious, well-rounded diet.

2.1. The Value of a Well-Balanced Diet

The importance of eating a balanced diet is often undervalued in our fast-paced society. A balanced diet is essential to leading a healthy lifestyle, not merely a fad. This article examines the vital role that a balanced diet plays in providing your body with nutrition, promoting general health, and averting a wide range of health problems.

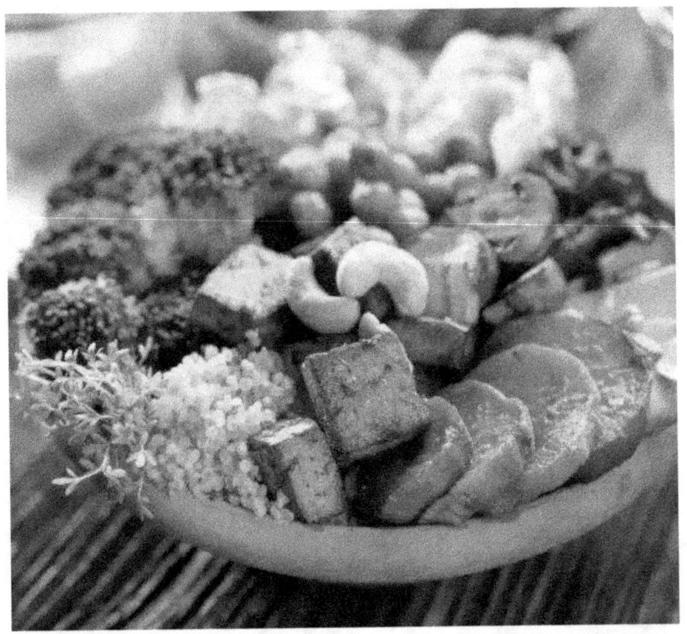

Important Elements of a Well-Blended Diet:

1. Basic Components: The body receives vital elements from a balanced diet, such as vitamins, minerals, proteins, fats, and carbs. Every nutrient is distinct and contributes to a different aspect of biological processes, such as immune system support or energy generation.

2. Balance of Energy: An adequate balance between calories taken and calories burned via physical activity is ensured by a balanced diet. Maintaining a healthy weight lowers the chance of developing chronic illnesses like obesity, diabetes, and heart disease, hence this balance is essential.

3. Prevention of Diseases: Eating a range of meals high in nutrients helps shield the body against sickness. A sufficient diet of vitamins and minerals boosts immunity, reduces vulnerability to illnesses, and improves general health.

4. Optimal Development and Growth:

Pregnant women, teenagers, and toddlers should especially follow a balanced diet. For the best possible growth and development as well as to avoid developmental problems, proper nutrition is crucial throughout these phases.

5. Cognitive Function and Mental Health: Cognitive function and mental health are directly impacted by nutrition. Rich in vitamins, antioxidants, and omega-3 fatty acids, a balanced diet promotes mental health, elevates mood, and lowers the risk of mental illnesses.

6. Stomach Health: Digestive health is promoted by a diet rich in fiber from fruits, vegetables, and whole grains. Constipation is avoided, regular bowel movements are facilitated, and a healthy gut microbiota is maintained by fiber.

7. Health of the Heart: A well-balanced diet that is low in trans and saturated fats lowers blood pressure and cholesterol while lowering the risk of cardiovascular disease.

Useful Advice for Maintaining a Balanced Diet:

1. Consume a Range of Foods: To guarantee a wide spectrum of nutrients, include a variety of fruits, vegetables, whole grains, lean meats, and healthy fats in your diet.

2. Control Point: Pay attention to portion proportions to prevent overindulging. Utilize smaller portions and pay attention to your body's signals of fullness and hunger.

3. Remain Hydrated: Drinking water is crucial to eating a balanced diet. Maintaining general health and supporting physiological systems requires staying hydrated.

4. Restricted Foods: Reduce your consumption of processed and sugary foods since they often lack important nutrients and, when taken in excess, may lead to health problems.

5. Make Ahead Meal Plans: To guarantee a balanced nutritional intake throughout the day, plan your meals. This supports you in choosing better selections and warding off the lure of quick, less nourishing solutions.

It is impossible to exaggerate the significance of a balanced diet. It is an effective tool for boosting general well-being, avoiding illness, and enhancing health. A road towards a better and happier life may be taken by those who adopt a balanced approach to eating, prioritize nutrient-dense foods, and make educated food choices. Recall that eating a balanced diet is about giving your body the nourishment it needs to flourish, not about going without.

2.2. Control of Portion

One of the most important components of keeping a healthy lifestyle is portion management. In a society where oversized servings and decadent meals are typical, knowing how to control portion sizes is essential for maintaining a healthy weight and avoiding overindulgence. This essay explores the benefits of portion management for your health, as well as its importance and realistic implementation tactics.

Why Portion Control Is Important

1. Control of Weight: Reducing portion sizes contributes to calorie intake, which is important for managing weight. You may avoid ingesting too many calories, which is often connected to weight growth and obesity, by eating the right amounts of food.

2. Norms for Blood Sugar: Stable blood sugar levels may be maintained with the help of proper portion management. Large servings regularly, particularly of meals rich in sugar or refined carbohydrates, may cause blood sugar to rise and fall, which can affect mood and energy levels.

3. Stomach Health: Overindulging in food may put undue stress on the digestive tract, which can result in pain and even long-term problems like acid reflux and indigestion. Controlling portion sizes promotes healthy nutrition absorption and digestion.

4. Conscientious Consumption: Portion management promotes mindful eating, which calls for paying close attention to what is being eaten. Understanding portion proportions encourages mindful overeating, allows you to appreciate each mouthful, and helps you identify when you are full.

5. Avoidance of Chronic Illnesses: Heart disease, diabetes, and hypertension are among the chronic ailments that are exacerbated by large portion sizes, particularly when it comes to bad diets. One proactive measure to avoid these health problems is to control portion sizes.

Techniques for Efficient Portion Management:

1. Make Use of Smaller Plates: Reducing the size of your plates might help you feel fuller after eating less by giving the impression that there is more food on them. It's a simple but powerful visual technique.

2. Apply the Plate Technique: Assign half of your plate to veggies, another quarter to lean protein, and yet another quarter to healthy grains. Appropriate portion amounts and a balanced diet are encouraged by this approach.

3. Be Aware of Your Body: Observe your body's signals of hunger and fullness. Eat mindfully, enjoying every taste and giving your body enough time to let you know when it is full. When you are pleasantly full, stop eating.

4. Weigh and Measure Food: To start, determine the right portion sizes using measuring cups, a food scale, or other instruments. Over time, this helps develop a feeling of portion awareness that may be used without instruments.

5. Avoid Being Sidetracked: Overeating might result from eating in front of the TV or while browsing through your phone. To better identify signs of fullness, concentrate on your food.

6. Primary Portions: Portion snacks into smaller containers rather than consuming them straight out of a big bag or container. This prevents careless overindulgence in food.

The ability to manage one's portion size is a crucial ability that enables people to make informed decisions about how much food they eat. You may attain a healthy balance, stop overeating, and enhance general well-being by implementing these tactics into your everyday routine. Recall that the goal is to cultivate a sustained and conscious attitude to providing your body with the appropriate quantity of food for optimal growth, rather than resorting to restriction.

2.3. Food Groups and What They Serve

The foundation of good health is a balanced diet, and making educated food choices requires knowledge of the major food categories and their purposes. Every dietary category provides a different combination of nutrients that the body needs to operate properly. We'll examine the main dietary types in this post and emphasize how important they are for maintaining general health.

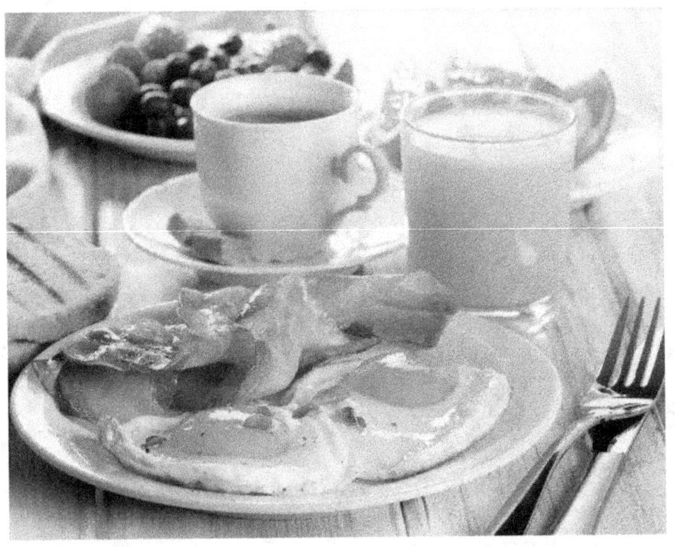

1. Veggies and Fruits:

- **Features:** Rich supplies of minerals (magnesium, potassium) and vitamins (A, C, and K).

- Rich in dietary fiber, which supports gut health and facilitates digestion.

Rich in antioxidants, which aid in preventing cell damage.

- Offer vital phytonutrients with possible health advantages.

- **Instances:** Carrots, spinach, broccoli, oranges, berries, and apples.

2. Grains with Carbs:

- **Features:** The body's main source of energy.

Packed with complex carbs that give you long-lasting energy.

- Has fiber, which facilitates satiety and aids with digestion.

- Provides minerals and B vitamins, which are vital for metabolism.

- Instances:

- Barley, whole wheat bread, quinoa, oats, and brown rice.

3. Foods High in Protein:

- **Features:** - Necessary for the development and maintenance of tissues, particularly muscles.

- Offers the amino acids required for a variety of body processes.

- Promotes the generation of hormones and enzymes as well as immunological function.

- Assists in controlling appetite and the sensation of fullness.

- Instances:

- Tofu, beans, lentils, seafood, eggs, and almonds.

4. Dairy and Dairy Substitutes:

- **Features:** - Excellent sources of vitamin D and calcium, which are vital for strong bones.

- Offers protein for the upkeep and development of muscles.

- Has additional vitamins (B12) and minerals (phosphorus) necessary for several body processes.

- Instances:

- Yogurt, cheese, milk, and fortified plant-based milk (almond, soy).

5. Oils and Fats:

- Features: - A source of vital fatty acids required for the health of the brain.

Facilitates fat-soluble vitamin absorption (A, D, E, K).

- Offers a focused energy source.

- Preserves the integrity of cell membrane structure.

- Instances:

- Avocados, almonds, seeds, olive oil, and fatty fish (mackerel, salmon).

Recognizing How Food Groups Interact:

- Correcting Macronutrient Balance

A macronutrient (carbohydrates, proteins, and fats) balance is necessary for a balanced diet to fulfill energy demands and support numerous body processes.

Diversity of Micronutrients:

Eating a range of meals from several food categories guarantees a varied intake of vital vitamins and minerals, which promotes general health.

Aqueous:

Water is essential for hydration and supports several body processes, such as digestion and nutrient transport, even though it is not a food category.

To achieve a diet that is both balanced and healthy, it is important to include a range of foods from several dietary categories. Specific nutrients from each food type are included and are essential for maintaining the body's operations. By being aware of the roles that different food categories play, people may make decisions that will best support their overall health and well-being. Always keep in mind that the cornerstone of a healthy lifestyle is a diverse and balanced diet.

2.4. Organizing Your Meals for Optimal Nutrition

Meal planning is an organized means of guaranteeing that your body gets the vital nutrients required for general health and well-being, making it a proactive method to attain optimum nutrition. This book examines the advantages of meal planning, offers helpful advice for efficient planning, and explains how it may help you meet your nutritional objectives.

The Advantages of Food Planning:

1. Nutrition in Balance: You may prepare meals that are well-balanced and include a range of dietary categories by using meal planning. This guarantees that you get the wide variety of nutrients—carbs, proteins, fats, vitamins, and minerals that your body needs to operate at its best.

2. Control Point: Meal preparation in advance facilitates good eating habits, quantity management, and the avoidance of overindulgence. It lets you split up how many calories you consume each day between meals and snacks.

3. Economies of Time and Money: You may cut down on food waste and simplify your grocery shopping by making meal plans in advance. This promotes more economical and thoughtful eating choices while also saving time and money.

4. Nutritious Snacking: Maintaining energy levels and avoiding unhealthy nibbling on processed foods are two benefits of including scheduled snacks in your daily routine. Having healthier alternatives on hand is ensured when you prepare healthy snacks ahead of time.

5. Alignment with the goal: You may match your diet to certain training or health objectives via meal planning. Whether your goal is to gain muscle, drop weight, or just maintain general health, organizing your meals around these goals can help you remain on course.

Useful Advice for Efficient Meal Planning:

1. Aim for attainable goals: Establish your dietary objectives while accounting for your lifestyle, degree of exercise, and unique medical requirements. Whether your goal is to lose weight, increase energy, or improve athletic performance, adjust your food plan to achieve these goals.

2. Develop a Weekly Menu: Make a weekly meal plan that includes a range of foods from several dietary categories. To add diversity to your diet, set aside particular days for different kinds of meals, such as a fish-based Friday or a vegetarian Monday.

3. Assemble ingredients ahead of time: To speed up the preparation of meals, wash, chop, and portion materials ahead of time. This facilitates speedier food preparation on hectic days.

4. Incorporate a Range of Foods: Make an effort to consume a wide variety of vibrant fruits, veggies, whole grains, lean meats, and healthy fats. This keeps your taste engaged and improves the nutritional composition of your meals.

5. Observe Portion Sizes: Learn about proper portion amounts by using measurement instruments. This aids in preventing overeating and improves your ability to regulate the number of calories you consume.

6. Take Nutrient Timing Into Account: Arrange your meals and snacks according to your activity level and daily routine. To promote energy levels and recuperation, make sure you consume an appropriate amount of nutrients both before and after exercise.

7. Swivel Recipes: Try different foods and switch up the recipes to keep things interesting. This adds diversity to your diet and keeps mealtimes from becoming monotonous.

Planning your meals is a great way to support your overall health and wellness objectives and achieve optimum nutrition. Planning your meals allows you to make deliberate, knowledgeable decisions that meet your dietary requirements. Recall that meal planning is an adaptable process, and maintaining a balanced and healthful lifestyle depends on discovering what works best for you.

Chapter 3. Examining Dietary Supplements.

The use of dietary supplements has grown in popularity as more individuals look for methods to improve their overall health and well-being. Good nutrition starts with a well-balanced diet, although some people use supplements to cover up nutritional deficiencies or take care of certain health issues. The fundamentals of dietary supplements, their possible advantages, use concerns, and the significance of making educated decisions are all covered in this article.

Comprehending Nutritional Supplements:

1. Explanation: A wide range of goods including vitamins, minerals, herbs, amino acids, enzymes, or other ingredients meant to complement the diet are referred to as dietary supplements. They are available in several formats, such as liquids, tablets, capsules, and powders.

2. Supplement Types:

- **Minerals and vitamins:** Vital nutrients that assist a range of body processes.

- **Herbal Supplements:** Plant extracts used in herbal remedies.

- **Protein Supplements:** Athletes often utilize them to aid in muscle building and recuperation.

- Omega-3 Fatty Acids and Fish Oil: Provides vital fatty acids for heart and brain function.

- Live microorganisms that support intestinal health are known as probiotics.

- **Amino Acids:** Protein-building components that are sometimes consumed to promote muscle.

- **Vitamin D and calcium:** Often administered to support healthy bones.

Possible Advantages of Nutritional Supplements:

1.**Deficits in Nutrition:** For people with certain medical issues or restricted diets, such as vegans, supplements may help make up for any nutritional shortfalls.

2. Dietary Specifics: Individuals adhering to certain diets, like veganism, may use supplements to guarantee sufficient consumption of particular nutrients that are not easily accessible in their diet.

3. Achievement in Sports: Supplements may help athletes perform better, recover from injuries, and increase their general endurance.

4. Particular Medical Conditions: particular medical disorders call for the use of particular supplements, such as calcium for osteoporosis or iron for anemia.

Things to Think About for Informed and Safe Use:

1. Healthcare Professional Consultation: It's important to speak with a healthcare provider before beginning any supplement program. Based on each person's unique medical requirements and possible drug interactions, they may provide tailored counsel.

2. Security and Quality: Select dietary supplements from reliable companies that meet quality requirements. Seek certificates from third-party testing to guarantee the effectiveness and safety of the product.

3. First, a Balanced Diet: A balanced diet should always be the primary source of nutrition. When feasible, try to get your nutrients from entire meals.

4. Amount and Time: Adhere to the suggested dose recommendations and consider when to take supplements—some work best when taken with meals.

5. Take Care When Using Mega-Dosing: Certain vitamins and minerals might have negative consequences if taken in excess. Steer clear of megadosing without expert advice.

6. Personal Requirements: When choosing supplements, take into account your age, gender, lifestyle, and specific health demands. What suits one individual may not be appropriate for another.

7. Avoid Additives and Allergens: People who have allergies or sensitivities should carefully read supplement labels to be sure no unwanted ingredients or allergens are present.

Although dietary supplements may be useful tools for promoting health, it is important to use care and consider each person's unique requirements when using them. While some people could benefit from taking certain supplements, others might get the best possible nutrition by eating a balanced diet. Recall that the safe and efficient use of dietary supplements depends on making educated decisions, speaking with medical specialists, and emphasizing a diet high in nutrients.

3.1. Addendum Categories

A vast variety of items intended to promote different facets of health and well-being are available from the supplement sector. Making decisions that support your health objectives requires knowledge of the many types of supplements. The main supplement categories, their functions, and factors to take into account when integrating them into a wellness regimen will all be covered in this article.

1. Minerals and Vitamins:

- **Intention:** - Complete any dietary nutritional deficits.

- Encourage vital biological processes.

- Support general health and welfare.

- Instances:

- Calcium, iron, magnesium, vitamin C, and vitamin D.

2. Botanical and Herbal Supplements:

- **Intention:** - Deal with certain health issues.

- Promote health using substances derived from plants.

- Conventional treatments for different illnesses.

- Instances:

- Turmeric for its anti-inflammatory properties; Echinacea for immunological support; and Ginseng for vitality.

3. Protein Additives:

- **Intention:** - Promote muscle development and repair.

- Offer a handy source of protein.

- Assist in the healing process for athletes or others who exercise vigorously.

- **Instances:**

- Whey protein; protein bars; plant-based protein powders.

4. Fatty Acids Omega-3:

- **Intention:** - Encourage heart health.

- Support the operation of the brain.

- Display anti-inflammatory characteristics.

- **Instances:**

- Fish oil pills, flaxseed oil, and omega-3 supplements made of algae.

5. Amino Acids:

- **Intention:** - The constituent parts of proteins.

- Encourage the growth and healing of muscles.

- Support a range of biological reactions.

- Instances:

The amino acids BCAAs (branched-chain), L-arginine, and L-carnitine.

6. Prebiotics:

- **Intention:** - Encourage the right mix of helpful microorganisms to support gut health.

- Assist with nutrition absorption and digestion.

- Support the immune system's operation.

- Instances:

- Bifidobacterium and Lactobacillus microorganisms in supplements or fermented food forms.

7. Performance and Sports Supplements:

- Intention: - Improve sports performance.

- Encourage recuperation and energy levels.

- Give nutrients suited for those who are physically active.

- Instances:

- Electrolyte pills, recovery beverages for after exercise, and pre-workout supplements.

8. Adjustments for Weight Management:

- Intention: - Promote weight increase or decrease.

- Encourage energy expenditure and metabolism.

- Offer nutrients to support certain dietary objectives.

- Instances:

Shakes that substitute meals, appetite suppressants, and fat burners.

Taking into Account When Selecting Supplements:

1. **Personal Requirements:** Choose supplements according to your age, gender, lifestyle, and personal health objectives.

2. **Expert Counseling:** Seek advice from dietitians or medical specialists to ascertain

individual requirements and possible drug interactions.

3. Security and Quality: Select dietary supplements from reliable companies that have certificates for third-party testing.

4. First Whole Foods: Give getting your nutrients from a balanced diet a priority before using supplements.

5. Amount and Time: Comply with the dose recommendations and take into account when to take supplements for best absorption.

Approaching the wide range of supplement categories with consideration is necessary. Although they may support a healthy lifestyle, supplements should be seen as an addition to a diet high in nutrients rather than as a replacement for it. Making decisions that support general well-being may be facilitated by being aware of the objectives of each supplement category and taking into account specific health requirements. Before adding additional supplements to your regimen, it's wise to consult a specialist, as with any health-related choice.

3.2. Minerals and Vitamins

A well-balanced diet must include vitamins and minerals, which are essential for sustaining health and supporting a variety of body processes. We examine the importance of vitamins and minerals, their sources, and their significant effects on general health in our investigation of them.

Knowing Your Vitamins:

1. Vitamins Soluble in Water:

- B-vitamins (B1, B2, B3, B5, B6, B7, B9, and B12) and vitamin C are two examples.

- **Functions:** Serve as coenzymes to assist immunological response, energy metabolism, and antioxidant defense.

- **Sources:** Lean proteins, whole grains, fruits, and vegetables.

2. Vitamins Soluble in Fat:

A, D, E, and K vitamins are a few examples.

Important for blood coagulation (K), bone health (D), antioxidant defense (E), and eyesight (A), among other functions.

-Sources: Leafy greens, nuts, seeds, fatty fish, dairy products, and seeds.

Unlocking Minerals' Power:

1. Electrical components:

-Instances: Magnesium, calcium, phosphorus, sodium, potassium, chloride, and sulfur.

-Functions: Essential for energy metabolism (phosphorus), muscular function (potassium), bone health (calcium), and several cellular activities.

- Sources: Whole grains, leafy greens, nuts, seeds, and dairy products.

2. Trace Elements (Microminerals):

- **Instances:** Manganese, iron, zinc, copper, iodine, and selenium.

- **Functions:** Crucial for immunological support, thyroid health, antioxidant protection, and enzyme activity.

- **Sources:** Fish, meat, whole grains, fruits, vegetables, nuts, and seeds.

The Effects of Excess and Deficiency:

1. Inadequate Vitamin:

Repercussions: May cause several health problems, including anemia (iron or vitamin B12 deficiency), rickets (deficiency in vitamin D), and scurvy (deficiency in vitamin C).

- **Prevention:** A diet rich in a range of nutrient-dense foods and well-balanced.

2. Deficiency in Minerals:

Repercussions: Inadequate levels may lead to ailments such as goiter (insufficient iodine), osteoporosis (insufficient calcium), and anemia (low iron).

- **Prevention:** A varied diet high in nutrients.

3. Excess of Vitamins and Minerals:

Repercussions: Overconsumption may result in toxicity, which can have negative consequences including sickness, damage to organs, or disruption of nutritional absorption.

- **Prevention:** Following suggested daily allotments and getting expert advice.

Making Well-Informed Decisions:

1. Well-Rounded Diet: A well-balanced diet that includes a range of fruits, vegetables, whole grains, lean proteins, dairy products, and dairy substitutes can help you get vitamins and minerals.

2. Extra Information: Speak with medical specialists before using supplements to treat certain health issues or deficits.

3. Recipe Techniques: Use cooking techniques like steaming or sautéing to retain the nutritional value of your meal.

4. Awareness of Interactions Between Nutrients: Recognize how different vitamins and minerals interact; for example, vitamin C improves the absorption of iron.

The hidden heroes of good health are vitamins and minerals, which affect everything from immunological response to energy metabolism. The best strategy to guarantee a sufficient intake of these vital nutrients is to adopt a diversified and nutrient-rich diet. By discovering the mysteries of vitamins and minerals, we enable ourselves to make decisions that support a happy, healthy existence.

3.3. Supplements with Herbs

The rebirth of interest in herbal supplements signifies a return to nature's healing embrace in a world where modern medicine rules. For millennia, people from many cultures have used herbal supplements, which are sourced from plants and botanical materials, for their therapeutic benefits. Nowadays, herbal supplements are becoming more and more well-liked due to their potential advantages as people look for natural alternatives to pharmaceutical medications and adopt a holistic approach to health. This essay delves into the realm of herbal supplements, illuminating their origins, variety, and possible health benefits.

Historical Origins:

Herbs have been used medicinally since the dawn of human history. Plants have long been known to provide therapeutic benefits in traditional medical systems including Native American herbalism, Traditional Chinese Medicine (TCM), and Ayurveda in India. This information has been handed down through the generations throughout time, and it serves as the foundation for many herbal treatments that are still in use today

Variety in Herbal Supplementation:

Supplements made from plants include a wide variety of plants and plant-derived materials. There is an enormous range, ranging from well-known herbs like ginger, garlic, and turmeric to lesser-known botanicals like ginkgo biloba, echinacea, and ashwagandha. Every plant has a unique combination of bioactive components that support its medicinal properties. Herbal supplements are highly customizable to individual tastes since they may be eaten in a variety of formats, such as capsules, teas, tinctures, and powders.

Possible Health Advantages:

The ability of herbal supplements to treat a variety of health issues is what makes them appealing. Certain herbs are well-known for their ability to reduce inflammation, which may assist with ailments like arthritis. Others have adaptogenic properties, meaning they help the body deal with stress. Antioxidants, which are abundant in many herbs, are essential in scavenging free radicals and lowering oxidative stress. Herbal supplements are also often utilized to boost immunity, support healthy digestion, and advance general well-being.

Obstacles & Things to Think About:

Despite the potential health advantages of herbal supplements, it's important to practice care while using them. Variations in the strength and quality of herbal supplements might result from the absence of conventional norms in the sector. Careful attention must also be given to possible adverse effects and interactions with drugs. It is important to speak with a healthcare provider before starting a herbal supplement regimen, particularly for those who are using prescription drugs or have pre-existing medical concerns.

Supplements containing herbs serve as a link between traditional medicine and contemporary health. These herbal treatments provide a natural and comprehensive approach to health at a time when people are looking for alternatives to traditional medicine more and more. Herbal supplements are a fascinating and varied field, but it's important to exercise caution and awareness while using them. Realizing the possible advantages of herbal supplements may be a start toward living a more balanced, healthier life with the correct knowledge and assistance.

3.4. Athletics and Enhancers of Performance

Athletes and fitness enthusiasts often experiment with different approaches to improve their performance in the quest for athletic greatness. People are looking for methods to exceed their physical boundaries, which has led to a spike in popularity in the sports and performance-enhancement industries. This article explores the world of sports and performance enhancers, including everything from legal supplements to contentious drugs, and it clarifies the benefits, drawbacks, and moral dilemmas related to these goods.

Enhancers of Legal Performance:

1. Dietary Supplements: Protein powders, amino acids, and vitamins are examples of nutritional supplements that are the cornerstone of lawful performance enhancement. The purpose of these supplements is to promote general health, recuperation, and muscular development. They are often used by athletes to maximize their training results and cover nutritional deficits.

2.   Creatine: One naturally occurring substance that is essential to the synthesis of energy is creatine. Creatine has been shown to increase muscular growth, strength, and power. It is generally acknowledged as a safe and effective supplement. It's a common option for athletes that participate in quick, high-intensity workouts.

3. Coffee: Caffeine is a stimulant that may be found in coffee, tea, and certain supplements. It is known to increase attention, alertness, and endurance. Caffeine is often used strategically by athletes to improve their performance during practice or competition.

Contentious Enhancers of Performance:

1. Steroids for Anabolism: Synthetic drugs called anabolic steroids work similarly to testosterone to increase muscle mass and strength. Although they may improve sports performance, using them has significant health risks and raises ethical questions. Hormonal imbalances, cardiovascular problems, and long-term organ damage may result from abusing steroids.

2. HGH (Human Growth Hormone): Growth and development are regulated by the hormone HGH. Synthetic HGH is used by certain sportsmen to promote muscle development and enhance recuperation. On the other hand, overuse of HGH may lead to negative consequences including insulin resistance, fluid retention, and joint discomfort.

3. EPO (erythropoietin): The hormone EPO increases the ability of red blood cells to transport oxygen by stimulating their synthesis. EPO is used by athletes, especially those in endurance sports, to increase their stamina. Abuse may raise hematocrit levels, which can put patients at risk for dangerous conditions including stroke and blood clotting.

Moral Aspects to Take into Account:

There are moral concerns about fair play, health, and the integrity of sports when performance enhancers are used. Strict rules are enforced by anti-doping authorities and sports organizations to preserve fair competition and safeguard the health of athletes. Athletes are advised to weigh the possible repercussions of utilizing prohibited drugs while giving preference to safe, natural means of enhancing performance.

Reaching top performance in athletics is a difficult path that requires commitment, self-control, and moral reflection. Legal performance enhancers may provide athletes a real advantage, but using these dubious drugs carries serious hazards for one's health as well as the integrity of competition. Maintaining integrity while enhancing performance is essential for athletes looking to succeed in their chosen fields over the long term. The complex world of sports and performance enhancers requires careful consideration of the importance of ethics, openness, and education.

3.5. Supplements' Place in a Healthy Lifestyle

People who want to be as healthy as possible often combine a healthy diet, frequent exercise, and enough sleep. While eating whole foods is the best way to receive important nutrients, meeting all of one's nutritional requirements may sometimes be difficult due to contemporary lifestyles and dietary choices. Here's when dietary supplements come in handy. This article examines the role that supplements play in completing nutritional gaps and promoting a healthy lifestyle.

1. Deficiencies in Nutrients: Even with our best attempts to have a well-rounded diet, deficits in some nutrients may nevertheless arise. Gaps in critical nutrients may be caused by a variety of factors, including food processing, soil depletion, and personal dietary constraints. To remedy these shortages and make sure the body gets the essential vitamins, minerals, and other components, supplements provide a practical and efficient solution.

2. Affordability and Availability: Fast-paced lives and hectic schedules might result in less-than-ideal eating habits in today's fast-paced society. Supplements are a practical answer since they are readily ingested concentrated sources of nutrients in the shape of liquids, pills, capsules, or powders. People find it simpler to keep their nutritional balance even during busy times because of this accessibility.

3.   Intended   Health   Objectives: Supplements to the diet might be customized to meet certain health objectives. There are supplements made to target different areas of well-being, such as stronger joints, better immune system function, or enhanced cognitive function. For instance, probiotics may help maintain a healthy gut microbiota, and omega-3 fatty acids may promote heart health.

4. Recovery and Athletic Performance: Supplements supporting performance and recuperation may be beneficial for those who regularly participate in physical exercise. Supplements containing protein assist in building and repairing muscles, whereas supplements containing electrolytes help replace nutrients lost via perspiration. Another such is creatine, which is well-known for improving power and strength during workouts.

5. Aging-Related Assistance: People may need different nourishment as they become older. When it comes to adding extra support for joint health, bone health, and cognitive health, supplements may be quite important. For example, it's usually advised to take calcium and vitamin D supplements to preserve bone density, particularly in older persons.

6. Encouraging Particular Diets: It may be difficult for those who adhere to certain diets, such as vegetarian or vegan lifestyles, to absorb certain nutrients from plant-based sources alone. In these situations, supplements may fill in the nutritional gaps and guarantee that people get the vital vitamins and minerals that they might not get from their selected eating plan in greater amounts.

Supplements are useful tools that, by correcting dietary shortages and supporting certain health objectives, may enhance a healthy lifestyle. They fill in gaps and support general well-being, but they are not a replacement for a balanced diet. It's critical to approach supplementing with knowledge and individuality, speaking with medical specialists to ascertain specific requirements and making sure supplements are included in a comprehensive strategy for a long and healthy life.

3.6. When & Why to Take Supplements Into Account

A well-balanced diet is the cornerstone of the path to optimum health. Even while we do our hardest to maintain a healthy diet, there are times when our bodies may need a little more assistance. This is the role of dietary supplements. This article examines the situations when taking supplements into account is advantageous as well as the rationale for combining them into a holistic approach to wellness.

1. Deficiencies in Nutrients: A major factor to take into account when thinking about supplements is the existence of nutritional deficits. Inadequate consumption of vital vitamins and minerals may result from several circumstances, such as dietary limitations, restricted food options, or certain medical disorders. Frequent blood tests and physical examinations may assist in detecting deficiencies, which can then inform the focused use of supplements to close these nutritional gaps.

2. Hectic Lives: A continuously well-rounded diet may not always be possible in today's fast-paced lives. Those who have hectic schedules, travel often, or have restricted access to healthful, fresh foods may find it difficult to get all the nutrients they need from their diet. With supplements, you can make sure your body gets the vital nutrients it needs for optimum performance in a quick and easy method.

3. Remarkable Food Preferences: It may be difficult for those who adhere to stringent diets, such as vegetarianism, veganism, or other restricted diets, to receive certain nutrients only from food. Supplements may be a useful tool to support these dietary decisions and guarantee that people get essential vitamins and minerals that may be in lower quantities in their selected eating regimens.

4. Recovery and Athletic Performance: Frequent exercisers, particularly athletes, may need more nutrients than average. To meet these increased needs and maximize the advantages of exercise, supplements designed to enhance athletic performance and recovery—such as protein powders, amino acids, and electrolyte replacements—can be very important.

5. Needs Related to Age: Nutritional needs frequently alter as people age. Supplements may provide focused assistance throughout the numerous transitions the body goes through. For example, omega-3 fatty acids may support cardiovascular health, while calcium and vitamin D supplements may be advised to preserve bone health in older persons.

6. Tough Times and Immune Assistance: Supplements may provide extra support during moments of high stress or when the immune system may be weakened, such as during sickness or periods of heavy work. The body's natural defenses may be strengthened with vitamins like C and zinc, as well as herbal supplements with immune-boosting qualities.

Supplements are an essential part of any well-rounded diet, but they also cover a wide range of demands and enhance general health. A tailored strategy that takes into consideration lifestyle circumstances, possible nutritional gaps, and individual health objectives is necessary to understand when and why to seek supplements. Healthcare specialists may provide insightful advice that will guarantee supplement selections are well-informed, focused, and included in a complete plan for a more balanced and healthy lifestyle.

3.7. Typical Nutritional Deficits and Supplements as Fillers

Even with our best attempts to have a nutritious diet, there may be nutritional gaps that affect our general health. Dietary deficiencies may result from dietary restrictions, lifestyle decisions, or inadequate consumption of certain food categories. This article examines a few typical dietary deficiencies and how supplements might help close these nutritional gaps.

1. Calcium D:

*Common Dietary Gap:** Many people may be deficient in vitamin D, especially if they don't get much sun exposure or live in an area with little sunshine. This vital vitamin is important for immune system performance, bone health, and general well-being.

***Supplement Solution:** Deficiencies may be addressed with vitamin D supplements, which are often in the form of vitamin D3. Appropriate supplementation may be guided by routine blood level monitoring and consultation with healthcare specialists.

2. Iron:

***Common Dietary Gap:** People with restricted diets and women of reproductive age are particularly susceptible to iron insufficiency. Weakness, weariness, and anemia may result from inadequate iron consumption.

***Supplement Solution:** Supplementing with iron may help restore iron reserves. They can be taken on their own or in combination with multivitamins. Nevertheless, consuming too much iron might have negative consequences, which highlights the need for expert advice.

3. Calcium:

***Common Dietary Gap:** People who are lactose intolerant or follow a diet that excludes dairy products may not get enough calcium, which is essential for healthy bones and muscles.

***Supplement Solution**: The body can get the calcium it needs from supplements if it also gets vitamin D for better absorption. Important factors to take into account include dietary modifications and speaking with medical professionals.

4. Fatty Acids Omega-3:

***Common Dietary Gap:** Inadequate intake of these vital fatty acids may hurt cognitive and cardiovascular health when diets deficient in fatty fish and plant-based omega-3 sources are followed.

***Supplement Solution:** A simple approach to guarantee sufficient omega-3 consumption is to take omega-3 supplements, including fish oil or algae-based supplements for vegetarians.

5. B12 vitamin:

***Common Dietary Gap:** Since animal products are the main source of vitamin B12, those who eat a vegetarian or vegan diet may not obtain enough of it. A B12 shortage may cause anemia, weariness, and nerve damage.

***Supplement Solution:** Foods enriched with vitamin B12 or supplements may help close this gap. For those with dietary limitations, it is essential to get expert guidance and conduct routine monitoring.

6. Isodine:

***Common Dietary Gap:** Diets low in iodized salt and seafood may be deficient in iodine, which is necessary for thyroid function.

***Supplement Solution:** You may avoid deficits by including iodine-rich meals or taking supplements. Nonetheless, it's best to prevent overindulging, and speaking with medical professionals is advised.

Resolving common dietary deficiencies is crucial to preserving good health. Although the best way to get nutrients is via entire meals, supplements might help address some dietary gaps. To guarantee that supplements are taken responsibly and customized to each person's requirements, professional assistance is essential to promote a thorough and well-rounded approach to nutritional well-being.

Chapter 4: Getting Around the Superfood World

The phrase "superfoods" has gained popularity in the field of nutrition, drawing interest from both foodies and health enthusiasts. These nutrient-dense marvels are praised for their extraordinary health advantages and high levels of antioxidants, vitamins, and minerals. This investigation reveals the nutritional powerhouses that may improve our diets and enhance our general well-being as we set out to navigate the world of superfoods.

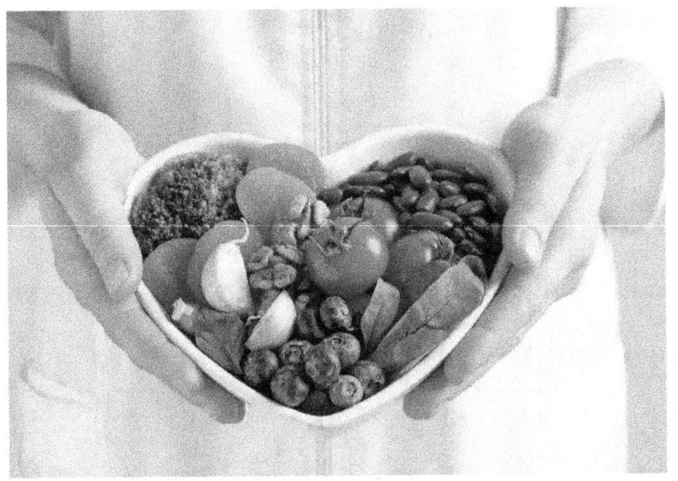

1. What is a Superfood? The word "superfood" refers to very nutrient-dense foods; it is not a categorization used in science. These meals contain a variety of health-promoting substances that may have a good effect on different body processes, going beyond just providing basic sustenance. Superfoods are available in a wide range of shapes and colors, from colorful fruits and vegetables to seeds, nuts, and grains.

2. Filtered with Antioxidants: Because of their high antioxidant content, berries including raspberries, strawberries, and blueberries are often hailed as superfoods. In the fight against oxidative stress, antioxidants lower the chance of developing chronic illnesses and promote cellular health in general. These vibrant jewels are not only tasty but also adaptable, so you can easily use them in a variety of recipes, such as salads and smoothies for breakfast.

3. Vegetables with a high cruciferous content: Cruciferous vegetables like broccoli and Brussels sprouts, as well as dark, leafy greens like kale, spinach, and

Swiss chard, are nutritious powerhouses. These veggies, which are high in fiber, vitamins, and minerals, improve digestion, strengthen bones, and boost the immune system. They are perfect as a nutrient-dense side dish, in sautés, and salads because of their adaptability.

4. Flaxseeds and Chia Seeds Rich in Omega-3: Because of their high omega-3 fatty acid content, which is crucial for heart and brain health, chia and flaxseeds have gained a reputation as superfoods. In addition to being a good source of fiber, these little seeds help encourage regular digestion and fullness. Adding flaxseeds to smoothies or chia seeds to yogurt are easy ways to take advantage of their nutritious properties.

5. Curcumin Content of Turmeric: Curcumin, a strong anti-inflammatory substance, is responsible for the superfood status of turmeric, a spice that is often used in Indian cooking. Turmeric is a popular addition to health regimens because of its ability to decrease inflammation and relieve joint discomfort. Turmeric-based beverages like "golden milk" are a fashionable method to include this superfood in everyday meals.

6. Quinoa Packed with Protein: Among grains, quinoa is unique as a superfood because of its high protein content and comprehensive amino acid profile. Quinoa is thus a great plant-based source of protein for vegans and vegetarians. It is a mainstay in kitchens that are health-conscious because of its adaptability in salads, and bowls, and as a replacement for conventional grains.

7. Seaweed and Spirulina: Blue-green algae called spirulina is well known for having a high nutritious content, which includes protein, vitamins, and minerals. Spirulina, which is often taken as a powder or supplement due to its ability to strengthen the immune system and reduce inflammation, is regarded as a superfood.

Conclusion:

Discovering the world of superfoods invites us to investigate colorful, nutrient-dense foods that may improve our health and offer us a palette of nutritional options. Superfood integration may be a tasty and beneficial venture, but it's important to remember that nutrition is still primarily about diversity and balance. Superfoods provide a comprehensive approach to optimum health and vitality when paired with a balanced diet, regular exercise, and other healthy lifestyle choices.

4.1. What Makes Foods Super?

The phrase "superfoods" has been widely used in the constantly changing field of nutrition, often with claims of improved health and vitality. However, what precisely are superfoods, and how do they differ from the wide variety of available meals? The goal of this essay is to demystify the idea of superfoods by illuminating their properties, health advantages, and integration strategies into a well-rounded, balanced diet.

What Constitutes a Superfood?

The word "superfood" refers to foods that are highly nutrient-dense and rich in chemicals thought to have health advantages; it is not a term used in scientific categorization. These meals provide a plethora of vitamins, minerals, antioxidants, and other bioactive elements, frequently beyond the requirements of basic nutrition.

The attributes of superfoods:

1. Density of nutrients: Superfoods are distinguished by their high nutritional density, which denotes that they have a notably elevated concentration of vitamins, minerals, and other advantageous substances in comparison to their calorie composition. Because of this, they are powerful dietary supplements that don't contain too many empty calories.

2. Content of Antioxidants: Superfoods are known for having a strong antioxidant profile. Antioxidants are substances that aid in the neutralization of free radicals, which are erratic molecules capable of causing harm to cells. Superfoods can lower the risk of chronic illnesses and improve general well-being by battling oxidative stress.

3. Packed with Vital Nutrients: Superfoods are often excellent sources of vital nutrients that assist a range of body processes. These might contain minerals like calcium and iron, vitamins like A, C, and K, and healthy fats like omega-3 fatty acids.

4. Potential Advantages for Health: Superfoods may be good for your health, but they're not a miracle cure. For instance, berries high in antioxidants may help to boost cognitive function, while fatty fish high in omega-3s may promote heart health.

Examples of superfood

1. Redcurrants: Raspberries, strawberries, and blueberries are prized for their vitamins, fiber, and antioxidant content. They are adaptable and delicious both raw and frozen, and they may be used in a variety of recipes.

2. Verdant Greens: Powerhouses of nutrients, kale, spinach, and Swiss chard provide an abundance of vitamins, minerals, and fiber. They are necessary to maintain bone health, immunological function, and general vigor.

3. Seeds and Nuts: Superfoods like almonds, chia seeds, and flaxseeds are prized for their high protein, healthy fat content, and vitamin content. They are simple to include in meals and snacks and are great supplements to a well-balanced diet.

4. High-Carbohydrate Fish: Rich in omega-3 fatty acids, which support heart health, cognitive function, and inflammation reduction, include salmon, mackerel, and trout. Frequent fatty fish eating is advised for a well-rounded diet.

5.   Curry: Strong anti-inflammatory curcumin is found in the spice turmeric. It is recognized as a superfood due to its widespread use in culinary traditions and possible health advantages.

Superfoods: Including Them in Your Diet

Superfoods provide a wealth of nutritional advantages, but it's important to include them in the diet in a balanced, varied way. The body cannot get all the nutrients it needs from a single diet, underscoring the significance of a varied and comprehensive approach to nutrition.

1. Varietal Diet: A diet rich in a variety of colors and textures, with a range of fruits, vegetables, whole grains, lean meats, and healthy fats should be your goal. This guarantees a wide variety of nutrients, all of which work together to promote optimum health.

2. Diversity and Moderation: Superfoods may be beneficial additions to a diet, but moderation is essential. To optimize nutritional advantages and avoid over-reliance on a few select meals, include a range of superfoods.

3. Considerations for Individuals: When adopting superfoods, take into account dietary choices, specific health demands, and any pre-existing medical issues. Seeking advice from a dietitian or medical practitioner might provide tailored direction.

Superfoods provide an interesting new dimension to the field of nutrition with their high nutritional density and possible health benefits. Still, it's critical to see them not as isolated miracles but rather as a piece in a larger nutritional tapestry. People may take advantage of the nutritional benefits of superfoods and enhance their general health and energy by adopting a varied and well-balanced diet.

4.2. Nutrient-Rich Superfood Examples

Superfoods are becoming more and more well-known due to their remarkable nutritional profiles, which provide a concentrated dose of vital elements including vitamins, minerals, and antioxidants. Including these nutrient-dense foods in your diet may improve many elements of your health and general well-being. In this investigation, we will examine the particular advantages that superfoods provide while showcasing several instances of them.

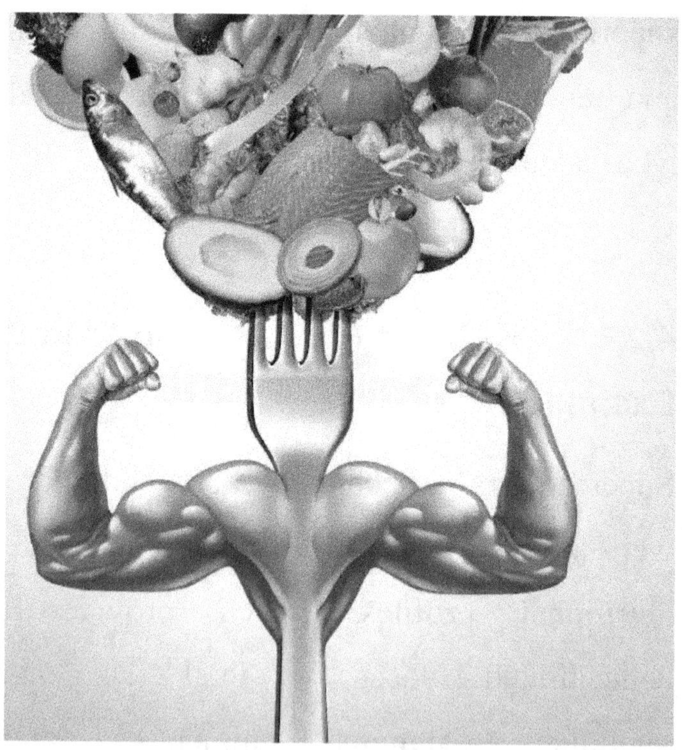

1. Redcurrants: Blackberries, raspberries, strawberries, and blueberries are a few examples.

Benefits: Packed with vitamins, fiber, and antioxidants, berries strengthen the immune system, promote heart health, and may even have anti-inflammatory qualities.

2. Verdant Greens: Swiss chard, collard greens, kale, and spinach are a few examples.

Benefits: Rich in iron, calcium, and other minerals, as well as vitamins A, C, and K, leafy greens support bone health, facilitate digestion, and provide a variety of antioxidants.

3. Seeds and Nuts: Nuts like almonds, walnuts, chia, flax, and hemp seeds are a few examples.

Benefits: Rich in protein, fiber, and good fats, nuts and seeds lower cholesterol, promote brain function, and aid in satiety and weight control.

4. A fish: Sardines, trout, mackerel, and salmon are a few examples.

Benefits: Packed with heart-healthy omega-3 fatty acids, fish also boosts brain function and may lower the risk of heart disease and other chronic illnesses.

5. Quinoa: Quinoa, for instance (pronounced keen-wah).

Benefits: Packed with fiber, vitamins, and minerals, quinoa is a complete protein source. It is a great substitute for conventional grains promotes the building of muscle and assists in digestion.

6. Yogurt from Greece:

Advantages: Packed with calcium, probiotics, and protein, Greek yogurt strengthens bones, promotes digestive health, and makes a filling and healthy snack.

7. Delicious Potatoes:

Advantages: Packed in antioxidants, fiber, and vitamins A and C, sweet potatoes improve immunity, strengthen eyesight, and may even help maintain good skin.

8. Curry:

Benefits: Turmeric, which is well-known for its main ingredient curcumin, has antioxidant and anti-inflammatory qualities. It may promote general joint health and lessen the symptoms of arthritis.

9. Broccoli:

Benefits: Broccoli is a cruciferous vegetable that is high in antioxidants, fiber, and vitamins C and K. It may have anti-cancer effects and promotes bone and immunological health.

10. Chocolate Dark:

Benefits: When ingested in moderation, dark chocolate with a high cocoa content may promote heart health and a happier mood since it is full of antioxidants and flavonoids.

Including superfoods that are high in nutrients in your diet may improve your overall health and well-being. These illustrations provide a wide variety of choices, enabling you to design a diversified and well-balanced diet that promotes general health. To fully benefit from these superfoods, it's crucial to keep in mind that a balanced diet is essential, and this includes a range of nutrient-rich foods.

4.3. How to Include Superfoods in Your Diet

Superfoods are becoming more and more popular as people look for better ways to improve their diets and general well-being.

Superfoods are foods high in nutrients, including vitamins, minerals, antioxidants, and other vital substances that support optimum health. Including these superfoods in your diet may help you feel more energized, strengthen your immune system, and lower your chance of developing chronic illnesses. This post will discuss the significance of superfoods and provide helpful advice on how to include them in your regular diet.

Knowing About Superfoods:

Superfoods are often praised for their remarkable nutrient profiles and possible health advantages. Several popular superfoods consist of:

1. Berries: Rich in antioxidants, vitamins, and fiber, blueberries, strawberries, and raspberries support heart health by lowering inflammation.

2. Leafy Greens: High in iron, calcium, and vitamins A, C, and K, spinach, kale, and Swiss chard help strengthen bones and boost immunity.

3. Nuts and Seeds: Rich in fiber, critical minerals, and healthy fats, almonds, chia, and flaxseeds support cardiovascular and mental health.

4. Fatty Fish: Rich in omega-3 fatty acids, which promote heart health and cognitive function, salmon, mackerel, and sardines are fantastic seafood options.

5. Turmeric: Packed with antioxidants and known for its anti-inflammatory qualities, turmeric also contains curcumin, which may ease several ailments.

How to Include Superfoods in Your Diet:

1. Make Minor Adjustments First: Start by including one or two superfoods in your daily meals. This gradual method facilitates a more bearable transition by giving your taste senses time to acclimate.

2. Juices and Smoothies: Blend your preferred superfoods to create mouthwatering drinks or smoothies. This is a handy method to mix different foods that are high in nutrients, such as seeds, berries, and leafy greens.

3. Combine with Salads: To add even more nourishment to your salads, add some berries, almonds, or seeds. A visually stunning and wholesome meal is created when bright fruits and seeds are paired with leafy greens.

4. Nutritious Snacking: Choose nutrient-dense snacks in favor of processed ones. Nuts, seeds, and dried fruits are nutritious and filling snacks.

5. Try Out Different Recipes: Investigate fresh recipes that use superfoods. To enhance the taste and health benefits of soups, stews, or curries, for example, consider adding turmeric.

6. Ingredient Substitution: Use superfood substitutes instead of less nutrient-dense products. For example, swap out rice for quinoa or add greens to your favorite pasta recipes.

7. Preparing the Meal: Plan your weekly meals and include a range of superfoods. This makes it more likely that you will continuously get the benefits of these meals high in nutrients.

Don't let superfoods intimidate you from including them in your diet. You may take advantage of the amazing health advantages that these foods provide by implementing little, long-lasting modifications to your dietary routine. Superfoods may add taste and nutrition to your everyday meals, whether your goal is to boost your energy, strengthen your immune system, or just feel better overall. Take the first step toward living a better lifestyle by realizing the potential of superfoods.

4.4. Recipes and Suggestions for Dinner

Taking a culinary trip makes every meal an enjoyable experience by opening up a world of taste and inventiveness. Whether you're an experienced cook or are just getting started, finding fresh recipes and meal ideas can liven up your kitchen. We'll look at a variety of dishes and meal ideas in this post that suit different palates, dietary requirements, and events.

1. Quinoa Breakfast Bowl:

Breakfast Bliss: A quinoa breakfast dish full of nutrients is a great way to start the day. After the quinoa has cooked, garnish it with sliced bananas, fresh berries, Greek yogurt, and chia seeds. For a delicious touch, drizzle with maple syrup or honey. Protein, fiber, and antioxidants are all well-balanced in this hearty meal.

2. Lunchtime Gem: Chickpea and Avocado Salad Wrap

Make a light avocado and chickpea salad for a pleasant and speedy lunch. Diced avocado, cherry tomatoes, cucumber, and red onion are combined with mashed chickpeas. Add salt, pepper, lemon juice, and olive oil for seasoning. Stuff this colorful combination into whole-grain wraps for a delightful and healthful lunch choice.

3. Supper Party: Grilled Salmon with Lemon Herbs

Salmon grilled with lemon and herbs can make a great meal. Marinate salmon fillets in a concoction of garlic, lemon juice, olive oil, and fresh herbs such as parsley or dill. Sear to perfection and serve with roasted veggies or quinoa. This meal offers a good supply of omega-3 fatty acids in addition to pleasing the palate.

5. International Flavors: Masala Chicken Tikka

Get your taste buds transported to India with a handmade masala of chicken tikka. After marinating chicken in a combination of yogurt and spices, bake or broil it until it becomes soft. Cooked chicken should be simmered in a tasty curry sauce made with tomatoes and served with naan bread or basmati rice. This rich and fragrant meal is guaranteed to wow.

6. Healthy Snack: Three Ways to Roast Chickpeas

Chickpeas that have been roasted are a crisp and filling snack. Toss chickpeas with your preferred flavor (cinnamon, cumin, or smokey paprika) and olive oil. Roast till crispy and enjoy a nutritious take on a common snack.

Trying out different recipes and meal ideas gives your cooking repertoire a more dynamic feel. These recipes offer you ideas for every meal, whether you're going for a gourmet supper, a full lunch, or a speedy and healthy breakfast. Accept the pleasure of cooking and let your palate discover the many options for delicious, healthful meals. Have fun in the kitchen!

4.5. How to Cook to Retain Maximum Nutrients

Cooking is more than just preparing mouthwatering dishes—it's also about maintaining the nutrients in the food. A lot of cooking techniques can cause food to lose vital nutrients. But, you can guarantee optimal nutrient retention and still enjoy tasty, filling meals by using a few deliberate techniques. To maximize the nutritional value of the ingredients in your food, consider the following helpful cooking advice.

1. Use Water Sparingly: Using as little water as possible is crucial when steaming or boiling vegetables. Vitamins that dissolve in water, such as B-complex and C, may seep into the cooking liquid. Use a modest quantity of water or steam veggies to reduce the amount of nutrients lost, and avoid overcooking.

2. Pick the Appropriate Cooking Technique: Some cooking techniques are more nutrient-friendly than others. In general, sautéing, steaming, and microwaving are preferable to boiling or deep-frying. By using these techniques, more vitamins and minerals are kept in the food.

3. Select Quick Cooking Option: Long cooking durations have the potential to degrade nutrients. To retain more of your food's nutrients, try cooking it rapidly. Stir-frying veggies for a brief period at high heat preserves their color, texture, and nutritional content.

4. Carefully Store and Handle Ingredients: The way you store and manage food might alter its nutritional value. Store fruits and vegetables in a cool, dark spot, and avoid cutting them too far in advance. Exposure to air and light might induce the deterioration of some vitamins.

5. Include Raw or Lightly Cooked Options: Incorporating raw or minimally cooked components into your meals might give an added nutritious boost. Some nutrients are more stable in their raw form, so try adding a side salad or fresh fruits to your meals.

6. Preserve Nutrient-Rich Cooking Liquids:

When you prepare foods like grains or beans, the water used in the cooking process may contain beneficial nutrients. Instead of discarding this liquid, try utilizing it in soups, stews, or sauces to ensure that the nutrients are not lost.

7. Avoid Overcooking Proteins: Overcooking meat, poultry, or fish may result in the loss of important nutrients. Cook these proteins only till they reach a safe internal temperature to keep their nutritious worth. Grilling, baking, or broiling are effective ways to keep nutrients in meats.

8. Appreciate Spices and Herbs: Use herbs and spices to make your food taste better instead of using too much sugar or salt. The antioxidant qualities of many herbs and spices may enhance the overall nutritious content of your meals.

By cooking with an awareness of nutrient retention, you may optimize the health advantages of your meals in addition to ensuring their deliciousness. You may eat tasty, nourishing meals that promote your general well-being by implementing these cooking suggestions into your daily routine. To achieve the ideal balance between flavor and nutritional content in your meals, try experimenting with various cooking techniques and ingredients.

Chapter 5: Customizing Diet to Meet the Needs of Each Individual

An essential component of maintaining ideal health and well-being is nutrition. Although conventional dietary recommendations provide a solid basis for healthy nutrition, it's important to understand that each person's nutritional demands might differ greatly. Personalized nutrition planning takes into account a range of parameters, including age, gender, exercise level, health issues, and genetic predispositions. This method not only improves general health but also helps in the management and prevention of several medical conditions.

Recognizing Individual Variations

1. Energy and Metabolism Needs:

Different people have varied rates of metabolism, which influences how their bodies turn food into energy.

- Age, body type, and degree of exercise all affect how much energy a person requires.

2. Hereditary Different:

- The way the body uses nutrition may be influenced by genetic variables.

- Due to genetics, certain individuals may be more prone to specific dietary deficits or intolerances.

3. Medical Conditions:

- Allergies, sensitivities, and chronic diseases may influence dietary decisions.

Certain dietary modifications may be necessary for conditions such as diabetes or cardiovascular disorders.

4. Activity Level and Lifestyle:

- More nutrients may be required by physically active people to maintain their energy expenditure and muscle repair.

- A different balance may be needed for sedentary lifestyles to avoid consuming too many calories.

Customizing Dietary Approaches:

1. Tailored Meal Schedules:

- Create customized meal plans that take daily calorie and nutritional requirements into account.

- Modify macronutrient ratios and portion sizes by exercise levels and health objectives.

2. Time of Nutrients:

- Take into account an individual's peak activity periods and modify nutritional consumption appropriately.

- Eating for exercise may maximize energy and recuperation.

3. Nutraceuticals and Functional Foods:

- Determine which particular foods, depending on dietary requirements, provide extra health advantages.

- Use nutraceuticals and functional foods to promote certain health objectives or to alleviate deficits.

4. Genetic Examination:

- Use genetic testing to determine dietary sensitivity or requirement predispositions.

- Adjust dietary suggestions by the genetic profile of the person.

5. Behavioral Aspects to Take Into Account:

When creating nutritional regimens, take into account cultural norms, personal preferences, and habits.

- Offer guidance and encouragement to people to adopt more sustainable lifestyles.

Advantages of Customized Diet:

1. Enhanced Absorption of Nutrients: People are more likely to efficiently absorb and use nutrients when their diets are tailored to meet their specific demands.

2. Prevention and Management of Diseases: By focusing on particular risk factors and nutritional needs, customized nutrition may aid in the prevention and management of chronic illnesses.

3. Improved Athletic Capability: By adjusting their diets to their training plans and activity levels, athletes may maximize their performance and recuperation.

4. Tailored Weight Control: Based on individual objectives, customized food regimens enable more efficient weight control by encouraging both muscle building and weight reduction.

Individualized nutrition planning is a dynamic, tailored method that takes into account the variety of human physiology and lifestyle. We can enhance general well-being, avoid illness, and maximize health outcomes by acknowledging and treating individual variations. Taking a customized approach to nutrition enables people to make educated food decisions that fit their own needs, leading to a more sustainable and healthy way of living.

5.1. Tailored Dietary Plans

The idea of customized nutrition has become well-known in the ever-evolving field of health and wellness as a ground-breaking method of enhancing personal well-being. Personalized nutrition, as opposed to universal dietary guidelines, customizes food plans based on each person's particular traits, such as genetics, way of life, and health objectives. This customized approach is a potent tool for improving general health and avoiding a wide range of health disorders because it acknowledges that every individual has unique nutritional demands.

Important Elements of Customized Dietary Practices:

1. Hereditary Elements: Genetic variants impacting nutrition metabolism may be identified thanks to advancements in genetic testing.

Comprehending genetic predispositions allows for customized dietary advice to target certain requirements and susceptibilities.

2. Difference in Metabolism: People vary in their rates of metabolism, which has an impact on the way the body breaks down and uses food.

- When determining the ideal macronutrient ratios and total calorie intake, personalized nutrition takes metabolic variability into account.

3. Deficiencies and Surpluses in Nutrients:

Evaluating each person's level of each nutrient makes it possible to pinpoint excesses or deficiencies and make exact dietary modifications.

This method helps avoid shortages that might lead to several different health issues.

4. Medical Disorders and Allergies:

Tailored nutrition provides dietary recommendations that improve general health by taking into consideration current health issues and allergies.

Personalized solutions are beneficial for those who suffer from illnesses such as food allergies, celiac disease, or diabetes.

5. Dislikes and Way of Life: Dietary choices, stress levels, and activity levels are all taken into account in personalized nutrition.

Personalized programs have a higher chance of being pleasurable and long-lasting, which encourages long-term commitment.

Putting Personalized Nutrition into Practice:

1. Evaluations of Nutrition: Carry out comprehensive evaluations that include health screens, lifestyle variables, and food history.

Employ cutting-edge technology to collect exact data for individualized suggestions, such as blood analysis or DNA testing.

2. Personalized Meal Schedules: Create individualized meal plans that take into account each person's dietary choices, calorie demands, and nutritional requirements.

- Take into account the timing of your nutrients to maximize energy and support certain exercise or health objectives.

3. Assistive Learning: Offer information and tools to equip people with the knowledge they need to make wise dietary decisions.

- Promote knowledge of how diet affects general health and well-being.

4. Continuous Observation and Modifications: Regularly assess each person's progress and modify the individualized nutrition plan as needed.
- Modify the strategy to take into account adjustments to objectives, health, or way of life.

Personalized nutrition's advantages

1. Maximized Uptake of Nutrients: People are more likely to efficiently absorb and use nutrients when their diets are tailored to meet their specific demands.

2. Enhanced Health Results: By targeting certain risk factors and nutritional needs, personalized nutrition may help prevent and treat chronic illnesses.

3. Improved Cooperation: Personalized nutrition plans enhance the chance that people will follow dietary guidelines, which supports long-term success.

4. Customized Weight Control: Whether the emphasis is on muscle building, weight reduction, or maintenance, personalized nutrition helps individuals achieve their objectives and promotes healthy weight control.

Personalized nutrition acknowledges and celebrates the individuality of every person, marking a paradigm change in the way nutritional recommendations are made. We can leverage the power of individualized dietary choices to support optimum health, avoid illness, and promote a meaningful and sustainable lifestyle by using a customized approach to nutrition. Adopting the tenets of customized nutrition enables people to set out on a dietary path that is as distinct as they are.

5.2. Nutritional Factors Affected by Genetics

Individual differences in dietary response are mostly influenced by genetic variables. Genetics and diet interact in a complicated and dynamic way that affects many elements of health, such as metabolism, nutrient absorption, and disease susceptibility. Comprehending these hereditary variables might provide significant perspectives on tailored nutrition strategies and assist persons in making knowledgeable food selections.

1. Thermogenesis and Energy Usage: A person's energy consumption and metabolic rate may be influenced by genetic differences. While some individuals prefer to retain energy as fat, others may have a stronger metabolism that enables them to burn calories more effectively.

- Differences in metabolism-related genes, such as those affecting the thyroid gland or adipose tissue, might affect the way the body uses and breaks down food.

2. Absorption and Utilization of Nutrients:

- Genetic variables affect how different nutrients are absorbed and used. For instance, some people may have genetic differences that impact how well particular vitamins or minerals are absorbed.

The efficiency with which the body utilizes food components may be influenced by genetic differences in the enzymes that are responsible for the breakdown and metabolism of nutrients.

3. Food Selections and Taste Preferences:

Taste preferences and dietary choices are also influenced by genetic factors. Some people's food preferences may be influenced by a hereditary predisposition to enjoy certain cuisines.

- Individual preferences for certain foods might be impacted by genetic variants that alter sensitivity to bitterness or sweetness, which may have an impact on total nutritional intake.

4. Allergies and Intolerances to Food: Food allergies and intolerances may arise as a result of genetic causes. People who have certain genetic predispositions are more likely to develop food allergies.

Knowing these genetic variables might assist people in recognizing possible allergies and guiding their decision-making to avoid negative responses.

5. Protection Against Disease Risk: An individual's vulnerability to certain nutrition-related disorders, such as obesity, diabetes, and cardiovascular diseases, is mostly influenced by genetic factors.

- Genetic testing and analysis may shed light on a person's susceptibility to certain illnesses, enabling tailored dietary and lifestyle changes as preventative measures.

6. Accurate Nutrition: Precision nutrition, in which dietary recommendations are customized to an individual's specific genetic profile, has been made possible by advancements in genetic research. Genetic differences are taken into consideration in personalized nutrition programs to maximize nutritional intake, enhance metabolic health, and lower the risk of disorders associated with nutrition.

5.3. Aspects of Lifestyle, Gender, and Age

In several industries, including healthcare, marketing, education, and social policy, it is essential to recognize and comprehend the many facets of age, gender, and lifestyle. These elements have a big impact on how people interact with the environment around them by forming their wants, preferences, and experiences. Acknowledging and implementing these factors is crucial in cultivating inclusion, customizing services, and advancing general well-being.

Age:

1. Stages of the Lifecycle: People go through many phases in their lives, and each has its requirements and difficulties.
Seniors may need specialized healthcare and community assistance, while children need caring settings and education.

2. Technological aptitude: The adoption and competence of technology are impacted by generational differences.
It's critical to adjust communications and services to the favored platforms and formats of various age groups.

3. Well-being and Health: As people age, their health needs change, underscoring the need for healthcare systems that handle age-related illnesses.

Encouraging preventative care and healthy lives becomes crucial.

Gender:

1. Identity of Gender: Establishing inclusive settings requires an understanding of and respect for the diversity of gender identities.

- Gender diversity should be honored and accommodated in policies and practices.

2. Impact on Socioeconomic Level: Gender roles may affect access to opportunities, wage levels, and job choices.

- Targeted initiatives in the areas of employment, social assistance, and education are needed to address gender-based inequities.

3. Health Inequalities: Disparities in healthcare access and gender-specific health concerns need addressing.

- It is crucial to adapt medical research and healthcare services to the demands of different genders.

Way of Life:

1. Cultural Diversities: varied ethnic origins may lead to varied eating habits, customs, and lifestyles.

Promoting unity and avoiding cultural insensitivity need an understanding of and respect for cultural variety.

2. Work-Life Harmony: Modern lives revolve around striking a balance between work and personal obligations.

- Workplace rules that facilitate remote work and flexible scheduling may improve people's wellbeing.

3. Integration of Technology: The rate at which technology is developing affects personal preferences and lifestyle decisions. Technology's impact on everyday life must be taken into account in several fields, including marketing and education.

Policy and Service Integration:

1. Designing with everyone in mind: Accessibility for a wider audience is improved by designing locations, services, and products with age, gender, and lifestyle factors in mind.

2. Targeted Marketing: Marketing tactics are more likely to resonate with the target audience when they are tailored based on demographic parameters.

- Inclusion is given priority in ethical marketing strategies, and prejudices are avoided.

3. Knowledge and Consciousness: Increasing knowledge of how age, gender, and lifestyle affect many facets of life fosters empathy and understanding.

- Educational establishments are essential in developing an inclusive culture.

To sum up, understanding the complexity of age, gender, and lifestyle is essential to building a society that is more inclusive and egalitarian. We may strive toward a society that respects and accommodates the variety inherent in the human experience by incorporating these factors into laws, programs, and daily encounters.

5.4. Diets with Specializations

Specialized diets have become effective tools in the ever-changing field of nutrition, helping to treat certain illnesses, optimize health, and accommodate personal tastes. These diets, which are often customized to meet specific demands, have grown in popularity due to their potential advantages and provide a complex method of fueling the body. Specialized diets are crucial in changing our perception of and relationship with food, from treating medical illnesses to improving general well-being.

1. Dietary Keto: Providing the Body with Fat.

Basis: - A high consumption of heart-healthy fats, a moderate quantity of protein, and a low intake of carbs define the ketogenic diet.

The objective is to get the body into a state of ketosis, which encourages weight reduction and mental clarity by switching the body's energy source from carbs to fats.

Uses: - Good for controlling certain neurological problems and losing weight.

- Research on its potential to treat diseases including type 2 diabetes and epilepsy is still ongoing.

2. Diet Based on Plants: Using Their Power.

Basis: - Whole, plant-derived foods such as fruits, vegetables, grains, nuts, and seeds are the focus of a plant-based diet.

- It may be embraced in a flexible manner, with varied degrees of inclusion of animal products, ranging from vegetarianism to veganism.

Uses: - Promotes heart health by lowering blood pressure and cholesterol.

Due to the less ecological imprint of plant-based diets, environmental sustainability is a motivating factor.

3. Diet Paleolithic (Paleo): Consuming Food Just Like Our Ancestors.

Basis: - The Paleo diet emphasizes foods including lean meats, fish, fruits, vegetables, nuts, and seeds that are thought to have been accessible to people during the Paleolithic period.

- Dairy, grains, legumes, and processed foods are not included.

Uses: - Proponents claim advantages including reduced body weight, increased vitality, and better regulation of blood sugar.

- The restricted nature of the diet and its possible effects on nutritional intake are issues raised by critics.

4. Mediterranean Diet: Indulging in Mediterranean Flavors.

Basis: This diet, which emphasizes fruits, vegetables, whole grains, seafood, and olive oil, is modeled after the customary eating habits of Mediterranean-coastal nations.

- Red wine, chicken, and dairy products should all be consumed in moderation.

Uses: Associated with better cognitive performance, a lower risk of chronic illnesses, and heart health.

- Acknowledged for being palatable and sustainable.

5. Gluten-Free Diet: Taking Care of Celiac Disease and Gluten Sensitivities.

Basis: Gluten is a protein present in wheat, barley, rye, and their derivatives. A gluten-free diet eliminates this protein.

- Crucial for those who have gluten sensitivity but do not have celiac disease.

Uses: Reduces symptoms in those with diseases associated with gluten.

In response, the food sector has expanded its line of gluten-free goods.

6. FODMAP Diet: Addressing Issues with Digestion

Basis: Limiting fermentable carbohydrates (FODMAPs), which are present in certain foods and may cause digestive discomfort in some people, is the goal of the FODMAP diet.

- Irritable bowel syndrome (IBS) and associated gastrointestinal disorders are often treated with it.

Uses: Provides comfort to IBS sufferers by reducing gas, bloating, and pain in the abdomen.

- Needs close supervision to provide enough nourishment.

Final Thoughts: Traversing a Customized Culinary Route

With their distinct uses and guiding concepts, specialized diets highlight the dynamic interplay between health and nutrition. Although these diets may be beneficial for some health issues, it's important to approach them mindfully and, if needed, seek advice from medical specialists or nutritionists. By adopting a personalized and well-rounded approach to nutrition, we may appreciate the variety of different diets and develop a healthy and long-lasting bond with our food.

5.4. Vegetarianism and Veganism

Examining Vegetarianism and Veganism: A Caring Lifestyle Option

The dietary practices of veganism and vegetarianism have become more popular in recent times. These decisions, which are based on moral, environmental, and health factors, signify a deliberate effort to rethink one's relationship with food. Adherents want to advance sustainability, lessen their influence on the environment, and adopt a compassionate lifestyle by abstaining from animal products.

Going vegan:

A vegan lifestyle abstains from all kinds of animal abuse and exploitation. This goes beyond nutrition and includes other facets of living including attire, makeup, and way of life decisions. But the main emphasis is on the diet side, where people avoid eating meat, dairy, eggs, and other goods that come from animals.

Motivations for Becoming Vegan:

1. Ethical Considerations: Concerns for animal welfare are a major factor in the decision of many vegans to choose this lifestyle. They don't support businesses that abuse or exploit animals because they think that animals should be treated ethically.

2. Environmental Impact: Many people believe that switching to a vegan diet is an ecologically beneficial decision. Pollution, greenhouse gas emissions, and deforestation are all directly caused by animal husbandry. By consuming fewer animal products, vegans seek to lessen their environmental impact.

3. Health Benefits: Some people decide to adopt a vegan diet because of the possible health advantages. Rich in fruits, vegetables, and whole grains, a well-balanced vegan diet may help reduce the risk of heart disease and several forms of cancer, among other ailments.

Going vegetarian:

Although vegetarianism and veganism both forgo meat, they differ in that vegetarianism allows animal products like dairy and eggs. Vegetarianism comes in many forms:

lacto-vegetarian (which includes dairy products), ovo-vegetarian (which includes eggs), and lacto-ovo-vegetarian (which includes both dairy and eggs).

Motives behind the Vegetarian Diet:

1. Health Considerations: To lower their consumption of meat's saturated fats and cholesterol, some people choose to follow a vegetarian diet.

2. Environmental Impact: Concerns about the effects of animal agriculture on the environment may drive vegetarians, just as they do for vegans. They want to help maintain the sustainability of the environment by cutting out meat from their diet.

3. Cultural or Religious views: People who follow vegetarian diets often do so because of their cultural or religious views, which promote kindness and non-violence toward animals.

Obstacles & Things to Think About:

Although vegetarianism and veganism have many advantages, those who are thinking about adopting these lifestyles should be informed of the possible drawbacks. It is important to make sure that sufficient amounts of vital nutrients, including protein, iron, vitamin B12, and omega-3 fatty acids, are consumed. Within the constraints of these lifestyles, keeping a healthy, balanced diet requires careful preparation and study.

Vegetarianism and veganism are strong decisions that take ethical, environmental, and humanitarian concerns into account in addition to one's health. A rising movement calling for a more thoughtful and compassionate approach to eating choices is fueled by people adopting these lifestyles, whether they are driven by concerns for animal welfare, environmental sustainability, or improved health. The importance of vegetarianism and veganism in promoting a compassionate and sustainable society is becoming more and more apparent as awareness grows.

5.6.   Gluten-Free   Foods   and Additional Dietary Limitations

A growing number of people have adopted different dietary restrictions in recent years for ethical, lifestyle, or health-related reasons. Gluten-free diets have drawn a lot of interest among these dietary options. The purpose of this article is to discuss typical dietary limitations and to go into the idea of living a gluten-free lifestyle.

1. Comprehending Diets Free of Gluten:

What Is Gluten? Proteins called gluten are present in wheat, barley, rye, and their byproducts. Those who have gluten sensitivity or celiac disease may experience inflammation and other health concerns as a result of ingesting gluten.

Gluten Sensitivity vs. Celiac Disease: While gluten sensitivity is a milder illness with comparable symptoms, celiac disease is an autoimmune disorder brought on by gluten ingestion. Both disorders need rigorous adherence to a gluten-free diet.

Gluten-Free Substitutes: The market has adjusted to meet the increasing demand for goods free of gluten. Common replacements include rice flour, almond flour, and tapioca flour. Furthermore, it is recommended to consume a variety of naturally gluten-free meals, including fruits, vegetables, and lean meats.

2. Extra Dietary Restrictions: Beyond Gluten:

Intolerance to Lactose: Lactose is a sugar that is present in milk and dairy products. People who are lactose intolerant lack the enzyme necessary to break down lactose. Dairy-free substitutes, such as almond milk or lactose-free goods, might be appropriate.

Veganism and Vegetarianism: Vegans cut out all animal products from their diets, whereas vegetarians refrain from eating meat. To guarantee adequate consumption of vital nutrients like iron, protein, and vitamin B12—all of which are found in large amounts in meat and dairy—these lifestyles must be carefully considered.

Allergies to Nuts: Nut allergies may be moderate to severe, and those who are allergic to nuts need to carefully avoid all nuts. It becomes important to read labels, and you may include other protein sources like seeds and beans.

Dietary Plan Paleo: The paleolithic diet, often known as the paleo diet, resembles the food habits of our ancestors. It usually entails avoiding grains, legumes, and dairy and eating lean meats, fish, fruits, vegetables, nuts, and seeds instead.

3. Guides for Managing Dietary Limitations:

Become Knowledgeable: It is crucial to comprehend the fundamentals of nutrition as well as the particular needs of the selected diet. Consult with medical specialists or qualified dietitians for advice.

Make Ahead Meal Plans: A balanced and fulfilling diet may be ensured by arranging meals in advance. Additionally, it may stop unintentional ingestion of prohibited substances.

Discover Fresh Recipes: Seize the chance to learn and try out new dishes that fit within dietary constraints. There are many tasty and inventive substitutes available on the internet.

Efficient Communication:
It's critical to communicate dietary demands clearly while eating out or at social gatherings. Many restaurants are accommodative and ready to change menu items to meet special requests.

Adopting dietary limitations, such as being gluten-free, may be liberating, but it takes thought and preparation. Through a conscious attitude to food selection and an appreciation of the subtleties of different diets, people may effectively follow these dietary routes and preserve their best health and well-being.

Chapter 6: Getting Around the Supplement Industry

In a time when wellness and health are major concerns, the supplement industry has seen unheard-of growth. There are a tonne of alternatives available to you whether you go into a health shop or explore online, many of which promise anything from increased energy levels to better cognitive performance. A discriminating approach is necessary to navigate this large and perhaps bewildering world. The purpose of this book is to provide you with the information and resources you need to explore the supplement industry with confidence.

Recognizing Your Needs:

It's important to determine your unique health and well-being objectives before wending your way through the sea of supplements. Do you want to strengthen your joints, strengthen your immune system, or improve your athletic performance? You may determine your specific requirements and make supplement decisions based on your needs by speaking with a qualified dietician or healthcare expert.

Quality Is Important

There are many different kinds of supplements on the market, and not all of them are made equal. Considerations for assessing a supplement include the brand's reputation, quality certifications, and independent testing. Seek for goods that have passed thorough testing to guarantee purity and potency and that follow good manufacturing principles (GMP).

Examine labels carefully:

Making educated decisions requires reading supplement labels. The component list, dosing instructions, and any possible allergies should all be carefully read. Furthermore, steer clear of proprietary mixes as it might be difficult to determine their effectiveness since they could not provide the precise quantities of each component.

Natural vs. Artificial:

Supplements may be made artificially or obtained from natural sources. While there are advantages to both kinds, some people want natural solutions. When choosing between natural and synthetic supplements, take into account your tastes as well as any possible sensitivities. It's important to remember that not all synthetic supplements are bad; in fact, some can be better in terms of consistency and purity.

Timing and Dosage:

To maximize supplement efficacy, timing, and dose must be correct. Ascertain the best time for your particular requirements by visiting a healthcare provider and adhering to the suggested dose listed on the label. While certain vitamins are better absorbed when taken on an empty stomach, some may be more effective when taken with meals.

Think About Whole Foods Initially:

Supplements are a useful adjunct to a healthy lifestyle, but a balanced diet full of real foods should always come first. A variety of minerals and phytochemicals found in whole meals combine to promote general health. A healthy diet should be supplemented, not substituted, by supplements.

Sifting through the supplement industry demands careful consideration and knowledge. You may make decisions that support your health and wellness objectives by being aware of your unique requirements, emphasizing quality, carefully reading labels, and starting with whole foods. Keep in mind that there is no one-size-fits-all approach when it comes to supplements, and speaking with medical specialists may provide you with individualized advice on your path to optimum health.

6.1. Selecting High-Quality Supplements

A plethora of products touting different health advantages might be bewildering when it comes to the world of supplements. We as customers must use discernment while navigating this market to make sure the supplements we choose are of the best quality and able to provide the desired effects. We'll go over important things to think about in this guide when choosing high-quality supplements to improve your health and well-being.

1. Testing and Certification by Third Parties: A crucial component of selecting high-quality supplements is making sure they are subjected to independent testing. reputable companies like NSF, USP, or

Informed Choice often do independent testing on their goods. These certificates attest to the product's compliance with strict quality requirements, attest to the correctness of ingredient labeling, and affirm that there are no contaminants present.

2. Transparency of Ingredients: Good supplements need to be completely transparent about what's in them. Look for labels that are clear and comprehensive, including every component and its exact dose. Watch out for proprietary mixes, which might obscure the precise proportions of each component and make it more difficult for you to determine their safety and effectiveness.

3. Surfactant and Strength: Seek for supplements that highlight potency and purity. A product's purity level indicates how free it is of pollutants like pesticides, heavy metals, and microbiological impurities. Conversely, potency guarantees that the supplement has a specified quantity of active components. Reputable producers conduct regular tests for these variables and publish the findings on their websites or product labels.

4. GMPs, or good manufacturing practices: Select dietary supplements from producers that follow GMPs, or good manufacturing practices. By guaranteeing that the goods are manufactured in a standardized and controlled environment, these procedures reduce the possibility of contamination and guarantee a constant level of quality. An indication of a manufacturer's dedication to quality and adherence to industry standards is their GMP accreditation.

5. Stomach accessibility: Take into account the supplement's bioavailability, or the body's capacity to absorb and use the nutrients. Nutrients may vary in their degree of bioavailability. For instance, the body may absorb certain vitamin forms and mineral chelates more readily than others. Do your homework on the bioavailability of certain nutrients so that you may choose supplements wisely.

6. Avoiding Dangerous Substances: Verify if the supplement contains any fillers, extra ingredients, or artificial coloring. Purity is the priority in high-quality supplements, and possibly dangerous ingredients are avoided. To reduce the chance of negative reactions, choose products with few, pure components.

7. Technical Proof: Seek supplements that have scientific support. Reputable companies fund clinical trials and research to back up their product claims. The product gains credibility and is more likely to have the desired effects when it is backed by scientific confirmation.

Selecting high-quality supplements is an essential first step in achieving optimal health and well-being. Third-party testing, ingredient transparency, purity, and potency are important factors to consider so that you may make well-informed selections that support your health objectives. Recall to speak with medical specialists if you have unique health issues or are unclear whether a certain supplement is appropriate for your particular situation. When carefully selected, high-quality supplements may be beneficial compliments to a healthy lifestyle.

6.2. Recognizing Labels

It might be intimidating to navigate the supplement aisle because of the rows of bottles with labels that promise different health advantages. It's critical to comprehend the information on these labels to make wise decisions. We will dissect the essential elements of supplement labels in this article to enable you to confidently interpret them.

1. Amount and Dosage of Serving: The quantity of the supplement that is regarded as one dosage is represented by the serving size. This information is important since it directly affects how many servings each container will hold. The recommended daily dosage of the supplement is specified in the dosage directions. To be sure you're reaping the desired results, carefully follow these suggestions.

2. The content of nutrients: To find out which vitamins, minerals, or other substances are in the supplement, read the section on nutritional content. Usually, the amounts are given in international units

(IU), milligrams (mg), or micrograms (mcg). Make sure the supplement is in line with the suggested daily amounts and your health objectives.

3. % Value Per Day (%DV): By showing the proportion of the recommended daily intake for each component in a single serving, the %DV gives context. This might assist you in determining if the supplement makes a meaningful contribution to your daily needs overall. Remember that your unique requirements may differ from the %DV, which is based on a normal daily caloric intake of 2,000 calories.

4. Additional Components: "Other Ingredients" includes ingredients like binders, preservatives, and fillers. Particularly if you have sensitivities or allergies, pay close attention to this area. To lower your chance of experiencing negative side effects, choose supplements with a few extra components.

5. Original Mixes: Proprietary blends, which are combinations of many components, may be listed on some labels. Even though certain combinations might have synergistic effects, the precise proportions of each component are often hidden. Proceed with care and, if at all feasible, choose supplements that list the precise dose of each component.

6. Information about Allergens: Look up information about allergens, particularly if you are known to be sensitive. Common allergies like gluten, soy, dairy, or nuts may be included in supplements. You may avoid goods that may cause allergic reactions by reading labels carefully.

7. Date of Expiration: Each supplement is guaranteed to stay stable and keep its efficacy for a certain amount of time, as indicated by its expiry date. Supplements that are consumed beyond their expiry date may become less effective.

8. Excellent Accreditations: Seek quality certifications from third parties that attest to the product's purity, potency, and quality, such as NSF, USP, or Informed Choice. These certificates show a dedication to production standards and provide confidence in the product.

Being aware of the information on supplement labels is essential to make responsible and knowledgeable decisions about your health. You can be sure that the supplements you choose are in line with your health objectives and uphold high standards by carefully examining serving sizes, nutritional content, %DV, and other important details. When in doubt, seek the assistance of medical specialists for specific guidance on the choice and dose of supplements.

6.3. Identifying Concerns and Red Flags

Although the supplement market is full of goods intended to promote health and well-being, there are certain issues and dangers to be aware of. Making wise judgments and avoiding dangers need the ability to see warning signs. We'll go over frequent disputes in the supplement industry and point out warning signs that buyers need to be aware of in this guide.

1. Unsupported Allegations: Supplements with ostentatious or unrealistic claims should be avoided. Although many supplements have a positive impact on general health, those that advertise instant cures or miraculous outcomes often exaggerate how beneficial they are. Seek for items that have scientific backing and promises backed by proof.

2.   Inadequate   Scientific   Support: Scientific research should be the basis of every credible supplement. Products without reliable clinical trials or research to bolster their effectiveness should be avoided. Producers who put effort into the quality of their goods are probably going to provide proof of their efficacy.

3. Secret Dosages and Exclusive Blends: Certain supplements use proprietary blends, which combine many components without giving precise amounts. It is difficult to evaluate the product's safety and effectiveness because of this lack of openness. To make educated selections, look for supplements that provide the dose of each component in explicit detail.

4. Too Much Stress on Marketing: Products with ostentatious packaging and gaudy marketing may prioritize appearance above functionality. Refrain from succumbing to advertising ploys and concentrate on the details on the label, such as component lists, dose calculations, and certifications.

5. Artificial Fillers & Additives: Check the ingredient list for any superfluous fillers, preservatives, or additions. Certain supplements include artificial sweeteners, colors, or flavors that might be harmful to your health or trigger allergic responses. High-quality supplements strive for ingredient lists that are clear and uncomplicated.

6. Inadequate Doses: Even while some nutrients are necessary for good health, taking too much of them might have negative consequences. Be mindful of the suggested daily intakes and steer clear of supplements that provide far more than is deemed safe. Excessive intake of certain vitamins and minerals may be harmful to your health.

7. Impractical Claims Regarding Weight Loss: Supplements for weight reduction are known for their audacious promises that are often unsupported by strong data. Products that promise quick weight reduction without requiring diet or activity adjustments should be avoided. Before adding weight reduction products to your regimen, speak with medical authorities.

8. Health Risks and Pollutants: Poor-quality supplements could be contaminated with dangerous microorganisms, pesticides, or heavy metals. Seek for items that have undergone safety and purity testing by a third party. Credible organizations' certifications, like NSF or USP, may attest to a product's compliance with exacting quality requirements.

9. Insufficient Regulation: Supplements are not subject to the same strict regulations as medications. This makes room for innovation but also lets inferior goods into the market. Select dietary supplements from reliable companies that value quality control and follow Good Manufacturing Practices (GMP).

6.4. Collaborating with medical professionals

Working together with healthcare providers is a great way to achieve maximum health and well-being. Supplements and lifestyle modifications may be quite effective in improving well-being, but professional healthcare advice adds a critical level of knowledge. This article examines the advantages of collaborating with medical experts and offers advice on how to create a cooperative and knowledgeable approach to your health journey.

1. Aware of Your Specific Needs: Physicians, licensed dietitians, and nutritionists are among the healthcare specialists with the skills and experience to evaluate your health profile. They may customize advice to fit your requirements by taking into account things like your lifestyle, medicines, medical history, and current **health issues.**

2.   Scrolling   Through   Supplement Options: The market for supplements is huge, and choosing the best ones may be difficult. Medical specialists may provide tailored advice on which supplements are safe for you based on your particular health state and in line with your health objectives. Additionally, they may assist you in avoiding any drug and supplement interactions.

3. Examining Laboratory Data: The findings of blood tests and other diagnostic evaluations may be interpreted with your assistance by medical specialists. Comprehending these results is essential for pinpointing regions that want improvement, recognizing dietary inadequacies, and formulating focused approaches to tackle certain health issues.

4. Determining Reasonable Health Objectives: Long-term success in health requires setting reasonable objectives. Medical specialists can help you set realistic goals based on your intended results and present state of health. By working together to create goals, you can make sure that your efforts are in line with your overall well-being.

5. Plans for Monitoring and Modifying: Because health is a dynamic state, you may need to make changes to your health plan over time. Visiting medical specialists regularly gives you the chance to assess your progress and make any necessary educated changes to your food, supplement regimen, or way of life.

6. Avoiding Possible Conflicts: Supplements and other medical treatments or drugs may interact. Healthcare providers can assist in identifying possible connections and reducing risks. Those who use prescription drugs or manage chronic diseases should pay special attention to this.

7. Assistive Learning: Healthcare providers are excellent teachers, offering knowledge about the science behind dietary supplements, lifestyle changes, and supplements. With this information, you may make more educated decisions about your health and develop a greater awareness of the consequences of those actions.

8. A Holistic Perspective on Health: Well-being is a broad notion that goes beyond dietary supplements. Healthcare practitioners use a comprehensive strategy, taking into account elements including physical exercise, emotional and physical well-being, stress management, and sleep. This all-encompassing viewpoint guarantees that therapies cover every aspect of your well-being.

6.5. Speaking with nutritionists and dietitians

Nutritionists and dietitians provide vital help in the pursuit of improved health and well-being. These medical practitioners are experts in comprehending the complex connection between diet, nutrition, and general health. This tutorial explains how getting individualized dietary guidance may improve your health journey and examines the advantages of speaking with dietitians and nutritionists.

1. Personalized Dietary Plans: Nutritionists and dietitians address your dietary demands on an individual basis. They may create customized nutrition regimens that meet your specific needs by taking into account things like your lifestyle, food preferences, medical history, and health objectives.

2. Managing Nutritional Inadequacies: Dietitians and nutritionists may detect any dietary imbalances and inadequacies via comprehensive evaluations. After that, they devise plans to fill up these deficiencies so that your body gets the vital nutrients it needs for optimum performance.

3. Healthy Eating and Weight Management: Dietitians and nutritionists provide evidence-based guidance on reaching and maintaining a healthy weight to those looking for assistance with weight management. Their advice goes beyond trendy eating plans and instead emphasizes long-term, balanced nutrition strategies that support overall health.

4. Taking Care of Chronic Illnesses: The knowledge of nutritionists and dietitians may be very beneficial to those who have long-term medical disorders including diabetes, heart disease, or digestive problems. These experts can create customized diet regimens to control symptoms, enhance general health, and support medicinal interventions.

5. Diet and Performance in Sports: Sports nutrition specialists may help athletes and fitness enthusiasts function at their best. To improve energy levels, recuperation times, and overall athletic performance, dietitians and nutritionists in this sector may design customized regimens since they are aware of the distinct nutritional requirements of different sports.

6. Teaching Good Eating Practices: As educators, dietitians and nutritionists provide information on the value of mindful eating, portion management, and a balanced diet. People are better equipped to make educated dietary decisions that improve their general health thanks to this educational component.

7. Emotional Eating Counseling: Nutritionists and dietitians may provide invaluable assistance to those who are battling disordered eating habits or emotional eating issues. To promote a better mentality and eating style, they provide therapy to address the root causes of harmful connections with food.

8. Management of Allergies and Intolerances: Dietitians and nutritionists may be of assistance to those who have dietary allergies or intolerances. These experts guide clients through dietary limitations, making sure that requirements are satisfied nutritionally while avoiding allergies or items that cause negative responses.

9. Promoting Sustainable Lifestyle Modifications: Nutritionists and dietitians emphasize long-term, lifestyle-fitting adjustments. Rather than pushing for extreme, temporary fixes, they collaborate with you to put into practice doable changes that you can sustain over time, promoting long-lasting health gains.

6.6. Interactions between Drugs

It's important to be aware of any possible interactions between supplements and pharmaceuticals as the use of dietary supplements increases. Supplements may have positive effects on health, but they may also interact negatively with drugs, compromising their safety or effectiveness. This article discusses the significance of understanding these interactions and provides advice on how to utilize supplements sensibly in conjunction with prescription drugs.

1. Interaction with Healthcare Experts: It's important to be transparent with your healthcare practitioner before starting any new supplement regimen. Tell them about all the medicines you use now, including over-the-counter, prescription, and dietary supplements. Healthcare providers may evaluate possible interactions and provide individualized advice using this information.

2. Possible Relationships: There are many ways that supplements and drugs might interact. While some supplements may improve a drug's effects, others may cause problems for the drug's metabolism or absorption. Reduced medication effectiveness or a higher chance of adverse effects might result from certain combinations. Interactions with blood thinners, antihypertensive drugs, and certain antidepressants are typical instances.

3. When to Consume It: Interactions may be affected by the timing of supplement and medicine use. While some vitamins work best when taken on an empty stomach, some may need to be taken with meals. The timing of an intervention may affect absorption rates and possible interactions, therefore it's critical to heed the advice of healthcare specialists.

4. Aware of Your Drugs: It is essential to comprehend the particular prescriptions you are taking. Certain supplement combinations may interact differently with different kinds of drugs. Vitamin K supplements, for instance, may have an impact on blood thinners, while calcium supplements may hinder the absorption of certain antibiotics. Making better-educated supplement choices is possible when you are knowledgeable about your meds.

5. Seeking Advice from a Pharmacist: When looking for information about possible interactions, pharmacists are excellent sources. Their comprehensive understanding of pharmaceuticals allows them to provide valuable perspectives on potential interactions between certain drugs and supplements. You may be educated about possible dangers and make well-informed choices regarding supplement usage by regularly speaking with a pharmacist.

6. Go Slow, Start Low: Starting with lesser dosages and then increasing as required is a good idea when starting new supplements, particularly if you are already taking medication. You may keep an eye out for any unexpected encounters or responses by using this careful attitude. Furthermore, introducing new supplements sporadically might assist in identifying the cause of any negative side effects.

7. Take Herbal Supplements With Caution: Herbal supplements may interfere with pharmaceuticals even though they are sometimes thought of as natural alternatives. Certain plants have strong physiological effects that might either enhance or decrease the effects of certain drugs. Inform your healthcare physician about any usage of herbal supplements you make.

8. Regular Reviews of Medication: Your pharmaceutical requirements may change as your health does. Treatment plan modifications are possible with routine medication evaluations with your healthcare professional. Now is a good opportunity to talk about any adjustments you may be making to your supplement regimen and look for any possible conflicts.

Chapter 7: Combining Exercise and Diet

A comprehensive strategy including many different components is needed to achieve maximum health and well-being, with activity and nutrition playing key roles. To improve energy levels, avoid chronic illnesses, and achieve long-term health advantages, these two pillars must be integrated. This material examines the mutually beneficial link between exercise and nutrition and offers suggestions for how people may easily include both into their daily routines.

Food:

1. Inner Body Sensation:

- A healthy lifestyle starts with a proper diet. Eating a well-balanced diet guarantees that your body gets all the nutrients it needs, such as proteins, lipids, carbs, vitamins, and minerals.

- Try serving your meals with a range of vibrant fruits, veggies, whole grains, lean meats, and healthy fats. This variety guarantees a wide range of nutrients that support general health.

2. Surfactant:

- Water is a vital yet sometimes disregarded part of the diet. Maintaining proper hydration promotes healthy digestion, maintains high energy levels, and supports several biological processes.

- Develop the practice of regularly consuming water throughout the day, particularly before, during, and after physical activity to replace fluids lost via perspiration.

Physical fitness:

1. Creating a Customized Exercise Program:

- Adjust your workout regimen to your tastes, objectives, and degree of fitness. A mix of cardiovascular, strength, flexibility, and balance training may be included in this. Take part in enjoyable activities to help you maintain a healthy lifestyle. This might be anything from yoga to team sports to hiking and dance.

2. Stability is Essential:

Frequent exercise not only helps control weight but also improves mood, lowers stress levels, and increases the quality of sleep. Maintaining consistency is essential for long-term health gains.

- Aim for at least 150 minutes of aerobic exercise at a moderate to high level or 75 minutes of intense activity each week, in addition to two or more days of muscle-strengthening activities.

Combination:

1. Nutrition Before Exercise:

- Two to three hours before working out, eat a balanced lunch or snack that contains both protein and carbs. This helps you perform at your best by giving your muscles the nutrition they need.

- Think about alternatives like a turkey sandwich on whole grain bread, Greek yogurt with berries, or a banana with peanut butter.

2. Nutrition After Exercise:

- Within 30 minutes after your exercise, replenish your body with a mix of protein and carbs. This replaces glycogen reserves and promotes muscle repair.

- A protein drink, quinoa-based stir-fried chicken and vegetables, or a fruit-yogurt smoothie are some of the options.

3. Be Aware of Your Body:

- Observe how your body reacts to various diets and workouts. Adapt your diet and exercise regimen to your demands, your energy level, and any health issues.

Combining exercise and diet is a great way to reach and stay at your ideal health. People may increase their energy levels, lower their chance of developing chronic illnesses, and improve their general well-being by making thoughtful decisions in both areas. Keep in mind that your health and quality of life may significantly improve with gradual, incremental, sustainable adjustments. Seek advice from dietitians or medical specialists to develop a customized plan that fits your needs and objectives.

7.1. Providing Energy for Your Exercises

Getting the most out of your exercises is essential to reaching your maximum potential, building endurance, and encouraging effective recovery. Whether you're a serious athlete or just a fitness enthusiast, knowing what to put in your body before, during, and after exercise will make a big difference in how fit you become overall. This article examines the role that a healthy diet plays in maximizing exercise efficiency and offers helpful advice on how to properly feed your body.

Nutrition Before Exercise:

1. Time is Crucial: - Giving your body a balanced lunch or snack two to three hours before doing exercise gives it the energy and nutrition it needs.

- Choose a balance of lean proteins and complex carbs. A banana with Greek yogurt, whole grain bread with almond butter, or oatmeal with berries are a few examples.

2. Hydration Is Important: Make sure you are well-hydrated before starting your pre-workout regimen. Exercise performance may be negatively impacted by dehydration and weariness.

- Have a glass of water every few hours throughout the day, and try to have an extra one or two hours before working out.

Nutrition for During Exercise:

1. Remain Hydrated: - Stay hydrated throughout your exercise by drinking water, particularly if you're working out for a lengthy or strenuous period.

- To replenish lost minerals and preserve fluid balance during prolonged activity lasting more than 60 minutes, think about consuming sports beverages that include electrolytes.

2. Short-Term Energy Increases: - For long-duration exercises like endurance training, ingest readily digested carbs to maintain energy levels. Energy gels, chews, or a little portion of dried fruit are a few examples.

Nutrition Following Exercise:

1. Recovery Protein: - Restoring glycogen storage and promoting muscle recovery occurs during the post-workout phase. After working out, eat a mix of carbs and protein within 30 to 60 minutes.

- Choices include a wrap with chicken and vegetables, chocolate milk, or a protein shake with banana.

2. Replace electrolytes and rehydrate: - If you've just finished an intensive or protracted workout, try consuming electrolyte-containing drinks in addition to water to help you rehydrate.

- To restore electrolyte balance, include meals high in potassium, salt, and magnesium. Bananas, oranges, and lush green veggies are a few examples.

Overall Dietary Advice for the Best Exercises:

1. Personalized Method: - Customize your diet to meet your specific demands, taking into account things like body weight, length, and intensity of exercise.

Try a variety of meals to see which ones suit your digestive system and yourself the best.

2. Level Up Your Macronutrients: - Strive for a diet that is well-balanced and rich in fats, proteins, and carbs. Every macronutrient is essential for promoting certain facets of your exercise regimen and general well-being.

3. Be Aware of Your Body: - Be mindful of signals of hunger and fullness. Adapt the amount of your pre-workout food to the time and level of intensity of your workout.

Maintaining general health and reaching your fitness objectives depend heavily on fueling your efforts. You can maximize your workouts, improve your recuperation, and perform at your best by taking a deliberate and personalized approach to diet. To ensure long-term success, keep in mind that consistency in your food choices and exercise routine is essential.

7.2. Nutrition Before and After Exercise

Making the right nutritional decisions is crucial to maximizing recovery during and after exercise and performing at your best. Nutrition is essential for both pre-and post-exercise since it helps your body meet the physical demands of exercise and recover from it. This article explores the significance of diet before and after exercise and provides helpful advice to help you make the best decisions and maximize the benefits of your exercise regimen.

Before-Workout Diet:

1. Combining Carbohydrates for Energy:

- The body uses carbohydrates as its main energy source. Eat a meal high in complex carbs two to three hours before doing exercise. This may apply to fruits, vegetables, and entire grains.

If you're pressed for time, have a smaller snack 30 to 60 minutes before going out. Choose simple-to-digest carbohydrates like peanut butter on a piece of whole-grain bread or banana.

2. Reduced Protein Consumption: - To promote muscular function, include a reasonable quantity of protein in your pre-exercise meal. You may include foods like plant-based proteins, yogurt, and lean meats in your pre-workout diet.

3. The Key is Hydration: - Drink plenty of water before working out. Throughout the day, sip on water, and think about ingesting 16–20 ounces more two to three hours before working exercise.

Steer clear of excessive alcohol and caffeine consumption since these substances might exacerbate dehydration.

After-Workout Nutrition:

1. Refuel Your Stores of Glycogen: - Your glycogen levels are reduced after exercise. After exercise, consuming carbs promotes recuperation and replenishes these resources. Select a blend of basic and complex carbs.

- Good options include sweet potatoes, quinoa, and fruit smoothies with extra protein.

2. Muscle Repair Protein: - Protein is essential for the development and repair of muscles. After working out, include a high-quality protein source in your meal or snack.

Lean meats, eggs, dairy products, and plant-based protein sources like tofu, lentils, and beans are among the options.

3. Recovery Hydrate: It's important to rehydrate after working out, particularly if you perspire a lot. To replenish fluids lost during exercise, sip water.

- To replenish electrolyte balance, if your workout was strenuous or extended, think about consuming a sports drink or coconut water.

Extra Advice:

1. Personalized Method: Try a variety of meals and timings to see what suits your body and tastes the best. Everybody has different nutritional demands depending on things like age, gender, and level of exercise.

2. Time Is Important: - To get the most out of post-exercise nutrition, try to eat a balanced meal or snack within 30 to 60 minutes after working out.

3. Extra Information: - Although the basis should be whole foods, if dietary demands are not satisfied, supplements may be taken into consideration. For individualized guidance, speak with a qualified dietitian or other medical practitioner.

Nutrition both before and after exercise is essential to a successful fitness program. You may improve your performance, lower your risk of injury, and promote optimum recovery by carefully selecting the ideal ratio of macronutrients and drinking enough water. Never forget that there isn't a one-size-fits-all strategy; instead, pay attention to your body's demands and change as necessary to reach your fitness objectives. Speaking with a nutritionist might help you get tailored advice for a diet plan that fits your particular needs.

7.3. Hydration Techniques

A vital component of general health, hydration supports a variety of biological processes as well as mental and physical functions. Creating efficient hydration plans is crucial, particularly for athletes, those with hectic schedules, and people who participate in physical activity. This material examines the significance of being well hydrated for good health, as well as symptoms of dehydration and doable tactics to prevent it.

The Value of Staying Hydrated

1. Body Temperature Regulation: The body's natural cooling process involves sweating. Sufficient water promotes efficient thermoregulation, which guards against overheating during exercise.

2. Transport of nutrients: Water is a transporter of vital nutrients, making it easier for cells to absorb them and supporting several physiological functions.

3. Memory Function: Cognitive functioning, including focus, attentiveness, and general mental performance, may be negatively impacted by dehydration. Sustaining appropriate water levels is essential for the best possible brain function.

Indices of Low Hydration:

1. Hungry: Feeling thirsty is a direct indication that your body needs extra liquids. It's important to remember that thirst is not always a reliable signal, since it may not always be obvious right away.

2. Dull Pee: Urine that is dark yellow may indicate dehydration. The urine of a well-hydrated person should be pale yellow.

3. Weakness and Vertigo: Dehydration may impair mental and physical performance by causing sensations of exhaustion, lightheadedness, and dizziness.

Strategies for Hydration:

1. Determine the Baseline: Assess your hydration requirements by taking into account your body weight, degree of exercise, and the local environment. Aim for 8 to 10 cups (64 to 80 ounces) of water per day on average, but make adjustments depending on your individual needs.

2. Regular Consumption of Water: Avoid depending on big quantities of water at once and instead drink water regularly throughout the day. Keep a reusable water bottle with you to make staying hydrated easy.

3. Balance of Electrolytes: To replace salt, potassium, and other minerals lost via perspiration, take into consideration drinking electrolyte-containing drinks during vigorous or extended physical exercise.

4. Remember to Stay Hydrated While Exercising: To determine your fluid losses, weigh yourself both before and after the workout. 16–24 ounces of water should be consumed for each pound lost when exercising.

5. Incorporate Foods That Hydrate: Eat foods rich in water content that are hydrating, such soups, vegetables, and fruits like celery, cucumber, and watermelon.

6. Modify for Altitude and Climate: The requirement for water is increased by environmental conditions such as heat and high altitude. When in hotter weather or at higher altitudes, adjust your hydration intake appropriately.

7. Restrictions on Dehydrating Drinks: Reduce your intake of liquids that might cause dehydration, such as alcohol and caffeinated drinks, since they can exacerbate fluid loss.

Drinking enough water is essential for preserving general health and enhancing mental and physical function. Well-being may be greatly enhanced by creating customized hydration plans based on individual requirements, routine monitoring, and conscientious fluid consumption. You can help your body perform at its peak and improve your capacity to meet the demands of an active and vibrant lifestyle by including intentional hydration into your daily routine.

7.4. Gaining Strength and Facilitating Healing

Enhancing muscle mass and facilitating recuperation are essential elements of any successful exercise program. Learning the fundamentals of muscle growth and recovery is crucial for reaching your fitness objectives and preserving your long-term health, regardless of your level of experience. This material examines important methods for combining exercise, diet, and lifestyle decisions to maximize muscle growth and recovery.

Developing Muscle:

1. Training in Resistance: - Make resistance training a regular part of your exercise regimen. This may include resistance band training, bodyweight exercises, or weightlifting.

- Pay attention to complex exercises like bench presses, deadlifts, and squats since they work many muscular groups at once.

2. Incremental Overload: - raise the complexity of the exercises, complete more repetitions, or lift heavier weights to gradually raise the intensity of your workouts.

- Gradual loading is essential for promoting the development of strength and muscle.

3. A Consumption of Protein: - Protein is an essential component of muscle. Make sure you consume enough meals high in protein to aid in muscle development and repair.

- Try to include some kind of protein in each meal, such as legumes, plant-based proteins, dairy, fish, poultry, and lean meats.

4. Time of Nutrients: - To maximize muscle protein synthesis and restore glycogen levels, eat a source of protein and carbs within 30 to 60 minutes after your exercise.

A protein shake, a well-balanced dinner, or a snack high in protein and complex carbs may all be good post-workout nutrition options.

Assisting in the healing process

1. Relaxed Sleep: - Give good sleep top priority to aid in general healing. The body produces growth hormone when you sleep deeply, which is necessary for both muscle development and repair.

- Try to get between seven and nine hours of sleep every night.

2. Surfactant: - Maintain enough hydration to maintain the body's general functioning, joint health, and nutrition transfer.

- Drink water continuously throughout the day, modifying your intake according to the temperature and degree of physical activity.

3. Nutrition in Balance: - Continue eating a diet that is well-balanced and emphasizes whole foods. A range of fruits, vegetables, nutritious grains, lean meats, and healthy fats should be included.

Foods high in nutrients provide the vital vitamins and minerals required for general well-being and healing.

4. Active Recuperation: - Include gentle exercises like yoga or walking on rest days to improve blood flow, ease soreness in the muscles, and speed up healing.

- Active recuperation maintains the body in optimum shape and helps avoid overtraining.

5. Mobility and Stretching Work: - To increase flexibility, lessen muscular tension, and avoid injuries, include mobility and stretching exercises into your daily routine.

- For general flexibility, it might be helpful to do static stretching after exercise and dynamic stretching before.

6. Be Aware of Your Body: - Keep an eye out for symptoms of exhaustion, overtraining, or discomfort in the muscles. To ensure adequate recuperation, modify the intensity and timing of your workouts as necessary.

Gaining muscle mass and promoting recuperation are linked activities that call for an all-encompassing strategy. Effective resistance training, healthy eating, enough sleep, and recuperation techniques all work together to create an environment that promotes muscular development and general wellbeing. Never forget that sustaining an active, healthy lifestyle and attaining results that last are mostly dependent on your ability to be consistent, patient, and sensitive to your body's cues. Seek advice from medical doctors or fitness experts to customize your strategy according to your unique requirements and objectives.

7.5. Consumption and Timing of Proteins

An essential macronutrient for many physiological processes in the body, protein is particularly important for muscle development, repair, and function. For anyone seeking to improve their fitness levels—whether it be for the purpose of developing muscle, enhancing sports performance, or maintaining general health—understanding the significance of protein consumption and when it should be consumed is essential. This material examines the importance of protein, daily allowance guidelines, and the best times to consume protein.

The Function of Protein

1. Growth and Repair of Muscles: - Amino acids, the building blocks of muscular tissue, make up protein. Gaining muscle mass and mending injured muscle fibers depend on consuming enough protein in the diet.

2. Enzymatic Processes: - Proteins are essential for many metabolic functions, such as the synthesis of enzymes, the control of hormones, and the operation of the immune system.

- A balanced protein diet promotes general health and keeps the body robust and functioning.

Suggested Daily Consumption of Protein:

1. Separate Variability: - Each person has different demands for protein depending on their age, gender, activity level, and fitness objectives.

- Many experts advise inactive people to consume 0.8 to 1.2 grams of protein per kilogram of body weight as a general guideline. Higher doses may be needed by athletes and those who exercise vigorously.

2. Active People and Athletes: - The amount of protein required by those who regularly engage in strength training or endurance exercises might vary from 1.2 to 2.2 grams per kilogram of body weight.

- To promote steady muscle protein synthesis, spread out your daily protein consumption equally.

Ideal Timing for Proteins:

1. Nutrition Before Exercise: - Two to three hours before an exercise, consuming a high-protein snack or meal supplies amino acids for energy and primes the muscles for the demands that lie ahead.

- A protein smoothie, a wrap with chicken and veggies, or Greek yogurt with fruit are some of the options.

2. After-Workout Hours: - The time after an exercise is crucial for muscle development and recuperation. Muscle

protein synthesis is maximized when protein is consumed 30 to 60 minutes after exercise.
- To restore glycogen storage, use a protein source together with carbs. A turkey sandwich on whole grain bread or a protein smoothie with banana and chocolate milk are two examples.

3. Protein Consumption Dispersed: - Spread up your daily protein consumption equally throughout the day rather to depending entirely on big, high-protein meals.
- Including a protein source in every meal and snack promotes overall nutritional balance and maintains muscle protein synthesis.

4. Just Before Going to Bed: - Having a high-protein snack before going to bed ensures that there is a constant supply of amino acids available throughout the nighttime fasting phase, which helps to minimize muscle breakdown and promote muscle regeneration.

Greek yogurt, cottage cheese, or a casein protein smoothie are among the options.

The right amount and timing of protein are essential for maximizing muscle development, repair, and general function. You may greatly increase your chances of building a strong, healthy body by adjusting your protein intake to meet your specific demands, exercise objectives, and daily routine. Whether you're a fitness enthusiast, competitive athlete, or just trying to maintain your general health, wise protein selection and timing should be important parts of your diet plan. Seek guidance from fitness or nutrition specialists for individualized recommendations based on your unique requirements and objectives.

7.6. Supplements for Recuperation

Exercise alone is not as important as post-workout recovery when it comes to achieving peak fitness and performance. Although a healthy diet, enough water, and rest are the cornerstones of recovery, several supplements may support these efforts and hasten the healing process. This article examines many supplements that have been shown to improve healing, lessen discomfort in the muscles, and promote general health.

1. Protein from Whey:

Role in Recovery: Leucine, which is important for the synthesis of muscle protein, is one of the necessary amino acids found in abundance in whey protein. After an exercise, whey protein consumption offers a rapid and effective supply of amino acids for muscle development and repair.

How to Use: For a quick and easy post-workout protein boost, mix whey protein powder with milk or water.

2. Amino acids with a branched chain (BCAAs):

Role in Recovery: BCAAs, which include valine, isoleucine, and leucine, are necessary amino acids that encourage the synthesis of muscle protein and lessen stiffness in the muscles. They are especially helpful for extended or vigorous activity.

How to Use: To promote muscle repair, BCAAs may be taken before, during, or after exercises in supplement form (capsules or powder).

3. Creatine:

Role in Recovery: A well-studied supplement, creatine improves power, strength, and muscle repair. It functions by restoring ATP, the body's main energy source, and minimizing the damage that exercise causes to muscle cells.

How to Use: Powdered or capsule form is the most popular form of creatine monohydrate. Take it once a day to help with muscular performance and recuperation, preferably after an exercise.

4. Fatty Acids Omega-3:

Role in Recovery: Fish oil contains omega-3 fatty acids, including EPA and DHA, which have anti-inflammatory qualities. They facilitate general healing, support joint health, and lessen inflammation brought on by activity.

How to Use: To improve absorption, omega-3 supplements may be taken with meals. Seek advice from a medical expert on the right dose.

5. Curcumin and Turmeric:

Role in Recovery: Curcumin, a strong anti-inflammatory substance, is found in turmeric. Turmeric or curcumin supplements may help to promote joint health, reduce inflammation, and ease discomfort in the muscles.

How to Use: Supplements containing turmeric may be bought as capsules or as part of a larger supplement that supports joints. For advice, speak with a medical practitioner.

6. Magnesium:

Role in Recovery: Magnesium is necessary for both the relaxation and proper operation of muscles. It could lessen discomfort, ease cramping in the muscles, and enhance the quality of sleep.

How to Use: There are many kinds of magnesium supplements. For improved absorption, think about taking magnesium citrate or glycinate.

7. Prebiotics:

Role in Recovery: Inflammation and general immune function are correlated with gut health, which is supported by probiotics. Better absorption and use of nutrients is facilitated by a healthy stomach.

How to Use: Select a premium probiotic supplement that has a range of strains. Regular consumption will help to support digestive health.

Supplements may speed up recovery, but they work best when used in conjunction with a comprehensive post-workout care plan. Make a balanced diet, plenty of water, and restful sleep your top priorities. Before adding supplements to your routine, think about speaking with medical specialists or nutritionists. Keep in mind that every person will react differently, so tailoring your strategy to your unique needs will help you get the most out of your recovery supplements for your fitness goals.

Conclusion:

Throughout the trip through the pages of "Powering Health: A Comprehensive Guide to Nutrition and Supplements," we have looked at the complex interactions that exist between the nutritional habits we follow on a daily basis and the substantial effects they have on our general health. This extensive manual sought to provide readers with the information necessary to make educated choices about their health by demystifying the complicated world of supplements and diet. It is crucial to consider the fundamental ideas that emphasize the significance of a diet rich in nutrients and well-balanced as we draw to a close this investigation. We have seen firsthand how decisions we make at the dinner table have a significant impact on our mental and emotional as well as physical health. The way that eating affects so many other areas of our life highlights how important it is to have a holistic approach to health.

We explored the importance of macronutrients and micronutrients throughout the book, comprehending their roles in sustaining essential body processes.

Every nutrient plays a unique role in the complex fabric of human health, from proteins that support muscle regeneration to vital vitamins and minerals that function as catalysts for many biochemical processes. With the ability to interpret nutritional labels, readers can now distinguish between goods high in nutrients and those low in calories.

We walked the tightrope between recognizing the possible advantages of supplements and stressing the need of a whole-foods-based approach while pursuing optimum health. Readers learned how to use these supplements wisely, making sure they enhance rather than take the place of a healthy diet. These supplements ranged from multivitamins to particular ones targeting certain health issues. The need for customized nutrition has also been emphasized in the book, acknowledging that every individual has different nutritional needs. Age, gender, activity level, and pre-existing medical issues are just a few of the variables that affect an individual's specific nutritional requirements. Accepting this knowledge gives readers the ability to customize their dietary choices to achieve their own health objectives.

As we get to the conclusion of "Powering Health," it is important to highlight how long this trip will take. Being healthy is a constant, dynamic process rather than a destination. The information conveyed in these pages acts as a compass, pointing readers toward the always changing field of nutrition. Making conscious and deliberate food decisions is a lifetime commitment to wellbeing rather than a passing phase.

"Powering Health" basically aims to motivate a paradigm change in our understanding of and regard for nutrition. It is an exhortation to see food as a potent instrument for building a robust and colorful life rather than just as a source of nourishment. The decisions we make now will have an impact on our health and energy in the years to come. Let this thorough guide's knowledge serve as a spark for revolutionary change, to sum up. May the ideas in these pages serve as a beacon of hope for long-term health and wellbeing, and may it inspire a love for feeding the body, mind, and soul.

Checklist of Nutrient-Rich Foods

Make sure your meals are nutrient-dense by using this checklist as a handy reference tool. Including a range of foods high in nutrients in your diet promotes general health and wellbeing.

1. Vegetables with Color: Add a variety of colorful veggies, such broccoli, bell peppers, carrots, leafy greens, and sweet potatoes. Various hues often represent various nutritional profiles.

2. New Fruits: Incorporate a variety of fresh fruits, such as apples, bananas, citrus fruits, and berries. Antioxidants, vitamins, and minerals are all found in fruits.

3. Complete Grains: Choose whole grains such as whole wheat, quinoa, brown rice, and oats. These grains include nutrients, fiber, and B vitamins.

4. Slim Proteins: Opt for lean protein sources including beans, lentils, fish, fowl, and tofu. Protein is essential for both general bodily functions and muscle regeneration.

5. Healthy Fats: Include foods high in avocados, nuts, seeds, and olive oil, which are good sources of fat. These fats aid in the absorption of fat-soluble vitamins and promote brain function.

6. Dairy and Dairy Substitutes: Add dairy products, or dairy substitutes enriched with calcium and vitamin D. Yogurt, milk, and fortified plant-based substitutes are among the options.

7. Dietary Probiotics: Foods high in probiotics, such as kefir, sauerkraut, kimchi, and yogurt, may improve gut health.

8. Fish: Add omega-3 fatty acids, which are vital for heart and brain function, by eating fatty seafood like salmon, mackerel, or sardines.

9. Seeds and Nuts: Eat a range of nuts and seeds, including flaxseeds, chia seeds, walnuts, and almonds. They provide vitamins, protein, and healthy fats.

10. Spices and Herbs: Use herbs and spices like parsley, cilantro, garlic, turmeric, and turmeric to enhance taste and nutritional value.

11. Aqueous: Water is the key to staying hydrated, which is the basis of good health. Try to have eight glasses a day or more, according on your own requirements.

12. Restricted Foods: Reduce your intake of processed and refined foods that are heavy in harmful fats, salt, and added sugars. Whenever feasible, go for whole, less processed choices.

13. Control Point: Pay attention to portion sizes to ensure that your intake of calories and nutrients is balanced.

14. Diversity Is Essential: To guarantee that you get a wide variety of nutrients, try to eat a varied assortment of meals. Change up your selections to include a variety of food categories.

15. Be Aware of Your Body: Be mindful of signals of hunger and fullness. Eating sensibly may help you make sure you're getting the nourishment your body needs.

You may prepare meals that are nutrient-dense, well-rounded, and support your general health and vigor by frequently crossing these components off. Make the most of this handy checklist to help you plan meals and shop for groceries so that you may maintain a healthy, well-rounded daily diet.

Guidelines for Supplement Dosage

To get the most out of supplements and minimize any hazards, it's important to make sure you take the recommended amount. To help you navigate the suggested doses for popular supplements, use this guideline as a reference. Before adding new supplements to your regimen, always get medical advice, particularly if you have underlying medical concerns or are on medication.

1. Multivitamins: - Take the daily dose as directed by the manufacturer.

- Select a multivitamin that provides a wide range of nutrients.

- Think about if you need to take any extra supplements based on your food and lifestyle.

2. Calcium D: - Everyday needs are different. For adults, general recommendations typically fall between 600 and 2,000 IU.

Speak with a healthcare professional to find out what you need in particular, particularly if you don't get much sun exposure.

3. Calcium C: - The usual recommended daily consumption for males is 75 mg, while for women it is 90 mg.

- For immune support, higher dosages (up to 1,000 mg or more) may be used at certain times, but first see a doctor.

4. Calcium: - Age and gender have an impact on adequate intake. Adults can need 1,000–1,200 mg per day.

Make sure you eat foods high in calcium, and if your diet isn't providing enough, think about taking supplements.

5. Fatty Acids Omega-3: - Dosage is based on personal health objectives. A typical dosage for overall health is 250–500 mg of mixed EPA and DHA.

Higher dosages could be advised for some ailments, such as inflammation of the joints or heart problems.

6. Iron: - Age and gender-specific daily needs differ. Men need 8 mg, while adult women may need up to 18 mg.

For those with iron deficiency anemia who have been identified, iron supplements are often advised.

7. Prebiotics: - Product-specific dosages differ. Observe the guidelines that the manufacturer has supplied.

- Take into account the particular strains and colony-forming units (CFUs) to get the desired results.

8. Magnesium: - Age and gender-specific recommended daily intakes differ. It might take 310–420 mg for adults.

- People with certain medical illnesses or inadequacies may benefit from taking magnesium supplements.

9. Zinc: - Age and gender-specific daily needs differ. While women only need 8 mg, adult males may need 11 mg.

Supplementing with zinc may be a good idea to strengthen the immune system or treat inadequacies.

10. B vitamins: folate, b6, and b12: - There are differences in dosages and individualized requirements based on medical conditions.

Sufficient food consumption is essential, and for certain groups of people, supplements could be advised.

11. Tautonym: - Doses vary. Commence with a modest dosage (0.5–1 mg) and modify as necessary.

Speak with a healthcare professional, particularly if you're using melatonin to help you fall asleep.

12. Chondroitin and Glucosamine: - Doses vary. As directed by the manufacturer. - When considering supplements for joint health, think about speaking with a medical expert.

Getting your nutrition from a well-balanced diet should always come first. A healthy lifestyle should be the foundation of any supplement usage, not the opposite. To maximize the advantages of supplementing, it is important to get individualized guidance from healthcare specialists since individual requirements may differ. A crucial component of appropriate and knowledgeable supplementing is routinely assessing and modifying supplement doses in response to evolving health requirements.

Dictionary

Explanatory

1. Antioxidants: - Materials that fight the body's oxidative stress by scavenging free radicals and minimizing cellular damage.

2. Stomach accessibility: - The degree to which a material or nutrient is taken up by the body and used after consumption.

3. Calorie: - An energy unit created from food that is used to calculate how much energy is in a meal.

4. Dietary Fiber: - Non-digestible carbohydrates derived from plants that support healthy digestion and increase feelings of fullness.

5. Enzyme: - Proteins that serve as catalysts for biological activities inside the body, enabling functions including metabolism and digestion.

6. Activists Without Labels: - Unpaired electrons in unstable compounds that have the ability to harm cells and accelerate aging and illness.

7. Gluten: - A blend of proteins included in wheat and other grains that give dough its elastic feel.

8. Shormones: - Chemical messengers that control different physiological processes and are generated by endocrine system glands.

9. Inflammation: - The immune system, blood vessels, and molecular mediators that are involved in the body's reaction to an injury or illness.

10. Small-scale nutrients: - Vital nutrients, such as proteins, lipids, and carbs, that the body needs in comparatively high quantities.

11. Minimum Nutrients: - Vital nutrients, such as vitamins and minerals, which are required in lower quantities to support different physiological processes.

12. Fatty Acids Omega-3: - Anti-inflammatory essential fatty acids, which are often present in fish oil and certain plant sources.

13. pH Equilibrium: - The body's acidity or alkalinity, which affects a number of physiological functions.

14. Prebiotics: - Live microorganisms, often bacteria, that are beneficial to health when ingested in sufficient quantities.

15. Additions: - Concentrated versions of vitamins, minerals, nutrients, or other compounds meant to be taken in addition to a diet.

16. Toxin: - Hazardous materials, which often refers to contaminants or chemicals, that have the potential to harm cells and tissues.

17. Complete Foods: - Foods that are unprocessed or just lightly treated while maintaining their inherent nutritional value.

18. Short-term Dieting: - Consistent weight loss and gain cycles, often accompanied by changes in body weight over time.

This glossary is intended to improve comprehension and encourage a deeper engagement with the material in "Powering Health: A Comprehensive Guide to Nutrition and Supplements." It may be used as a fast reference to define words that are used throughout the book. Feel free to go back to this glossary as you read through the content to confirm that you understand the important terms on nutrition and supplements.

9 798877 843103